MICU

The Guide to Residency

First edition

(This book is a reproduction of the original book "Internal medicine: The Guide to Residency" to include all the MICU related topics, with some additions)

Amer Sayed, MD
Georgia Regents University
Internal Medicine Resident

DISCLAIMER

Care has been taken to confirm the accuracy of the information presented in this book by reviewing the literature and books related to the subjects and by including the most common practice information and experience from the authors and editors stand of point . However, the authors, editors, and publisher are NOT responsible for errors or omissions or for any consequences from application of the information in this book and make no warranty, expressed or implied, with respect to the currency, completeness, or accuracy of the contents of the publication. Practitioners are responsible for applying this information into patient's care and the clinical out-come

The authors and editors listed the most common medicine and some of the doses used in practice according to their best knowledge, however, it is highly recommended to recheck the medicine indications and doses from an up-to-date source as they change with time. This is particularly important when the recommended agent is a new or infrequently employed drug. And it is the responsibility of the health care provider to ascertain the FDA status of each drug or device planned for use in clinical practice.

Contact the author by email:
internalmedicinetheguide@gmail.com

Table of Contents

CONTRIBUTORS

All are from Georgia Regents University

Contributing Authors:
**All are Georgia Regents University Residents &
contributed in the following chapters**

Eduard Fatakhov, MD
Haytham Alkhaimy, MD
Scott Graupner, MD
Abhishek Mangaonkar, MD
Gita Mehta, MD
Sasha Baker, MD

Contributing Editors:
Lee A Merchen, MD, FACP
Program Director, Internal Medicine Residency

James Gossage, MD
Division of Pulmonary/Critical Care
Professor of Medicine

Pascha Schafer, MD
Divison of Cardiology
Associate Program Director

Lu Huber, MD
Division of Nephrology
Assistant Professor

Gyanendra Sharma, MD, FASE, FACC
Division of Cardiology
Professor of Medicine

Thaddeus Carson, MD
Division of Internal Medicine
Assistant Professor

Meshia Wallace, MD
Internal Medicine Resident

Christina DeRemer, Pharm.D., BCPS
Pharmacy Supervisor, Clinical Service (Medicine)

Mike Garcia, PhD
Director of College Composition
Assistant Professor

Medical Students:
Danielle Bayer
Brandon Taylor
Evan Fountain
Amir Makhmalbaf
Zachary Hoffmann
Reshma Reddy
Kunal Patel
Nader Aboujamous

Medical Illustrator
Michael A. Jensen, MS, CMI
Assistant Professor

Special Acknowledgement
Walter J. Moore, MD, MACP, FACR
Division of Rheumatology
Professor of Medicine and Pediatrics

All GRU staff who provided assistance in this project

Preface

This guidebook is written to assist in the transition between medical school and internal medicine residency; it is designed to highlight the most common clinical cases presented and how best to manage them. The topics have been carefully chosen to cover common differential diagnoses to common symptoms. This book will give you a quick summary of what you need clinically to know about them as well as challenges you may encounter in the process. Ideally, this handbook can be read in 1-2 weeks and consulted at any time during residency, but especially during internship.

By reading this guide, written by current internal medicine residents, the reader will benefit from residents' actual experiences, both successes and missteps, which can aid the reader with patient care and case management. The guide includes managing the common clinical problems that patients are admitted for so the intern or the resident will feel confident and display more accuracy in examining the patient, obtaining medical history, writing a thorough and useful history and physical with appropriate work-up.

Unlike the other few available guide or pocket books, this one will NOT address unnecessary and hard-to-remember details you may NOT need in day-to-day practice in order to deliver the most high-yield information in short period of time. Since fourth-year medical students may have only one to two months of internal medicine training, they may become less familiar in managing common diseases after months of training in other specialties (NOT to mention the time traveling during match season and relocation takes). This book will prove to be efficient and effective even during this busy time.

The focus of this guide will be the common explanations for chest pain like acute coronary syndrome, pulmonary embolism; hyper/ hyponatremia, lower/ upper GI bleed, different types of pneumonia, atrial fibrillation, CHF, and so on. The primary resources and references we have used include *Harrison's Principles of Internal Medicine*, the *Washington Manual of Medical Therapeutics*, several published articles on internal medicine, and other resources. This book offers years of experience from residents and attendings, keeping you, a recent medical graduate, in mind. I must reiterate that the input of the attendings who took time to be a part of this project was crucial. This finished guidebook is a culmination of real clinical experience you will encounter presented in an easy-to-reference format written by the fresh perspective and experience of your fellow internal medicine residents.

Amer Sayed, M.D.
Internal Medicine Resident
Georgia Regents University

Foreword

As has been said by many, there is no greater privilege and no more challenging responsibility than to direct the care of those who are ill. More than knowledge, it requires competency, and more than competency it requires virtue, and more than virtue it requires both passion and compassion for another human being in distress. As an internal medicine residency program director for more than 25 years, it has been my joy to observe curious, empathetic, and disciplined students develop into wonderfully compassionate and consummate clinicians. They do this by focusing fully on their patients and their well being as men and women made in the Image of God, rather than data sets. Medicine is much more than making a diagnosis, prescribing a therapy, and offering a prognosis; it is a journey with another soul, sometimes for a shift, a day, a week, or decades.

Dr. Sayed's guidebook offers a convenient roadmap for the beginning of this journey. It is patient, rather than disease centered, and should be used as a starting point for the practice based learning and patient care competencies as well as virtues associated with hospital care and discharge planning. It is compact, convenient, and clear in its approach to the most common symptoms and problems of patients in modern hospitals.

Two things should be recognized by the reader, however: 1) Most hospitalized patients have more than one problem. They have multiple co-morbidities that include multiple diseases, social-economic, and especially psychological and even spiritual complexities that defy simple analysis and interact to thwart simplistic interventions. 2)

Situations in which patients find themselves are always dynamic and changing, with a past which may be hidden (especially childhood trauma and abuse), a presence which needs systemic understanding, and a future which depends on timeliness and follow through of plans made.

This reference is a fine start for the genesis of an outstanding clinician. Savvy students will initiate a lifetime habit of frequent and lengthy visits to both the bedside and the enlarging greater body of literature. In each location they will ponder deeply both the causes and the effects of what is happening to their patients. Then, with experience, time, and devotion, they will be able also to taste and give to others the fruits of their practice.

David R. Haburchak, M.D. FACP
Professor of Medicine
Georgia Regents University

Life is short and art long, Opportunity fleeting,
Experience perilous and decision difficult.
                    Hippocrates

1. Medical Intensive Care Unit (MICU)/Hypotension (HoTN)/Cardiac Arrest

Survival of the critically ill pt depends on initiating life-saving measures in a timely fashion. However, recognizing serious illness before the onset of overt instability can be challenging. For example, younger pts w/ sepsis can appear deceptively well but may develop multiorgan failure w/ in hrs. A systematic approach to pt assessment minimizes the likelihood of delayed recognition of critical illness.

The initial evaluation should consist of a brief bedside hx & focused examination to discern whether immediate action is needed to stabilize the pt's airway, breathing, or circulation. Review of vital signs over the preceding hrs often provides valuable information on the pt's overall current stability.

Common early interventions include intravenous fluid boluses for HoTN, O_2 & noninvasive ventilatory support for respiratory distress, & naloxone or dextrose (D50) for encephalopathy due to narcotics & hypoglycemia, respectively. Studies that may be useful for diagnosing the cause & determining severity of illness include ABG; CBG, Hgb, lactic acid levels, EKG, & portable CXR. Limited bedside TTE to assess the hemodynamic status of unstable pts has ↑ in recent years (i.e.: IVC compressibility).

After imminently life-threatening issues are addressed, a **more comprehensive secondary assessment** should be performed w/ an emphasis on identifying less obvious evidence of organ hypoperfusion. This includes AMS (confusion, agitation), ↓ urine output (<0. 5cc/kg/hr), skin changes (pallor, diaphoresis, cyanosis, cool extremities), & ↑ work of breathing.

Common indications for MICU admission
- Close nursing monitoring (example: unstable vitals for any reason like septic shock), service canNOT be delivered in the floor (like intubation & ventilation, arterial line for BP monitoring).
- Status post cardiac arrest & respiratory failure.
- The need for certain IV infusions (like labetalol, diltiazem, amiodarone, lasix, HCO3, etc).
- Sever physiologic changes (very low or high blood PH, severe electrolytes abnormalities like K, Mg, phosphate).
- DKA & HONK management (until the GAP closes & pt tolerate PO intake & get SQ insulin).
- Urgent /emergent procedures like EGD for (GI bleed) or dialysis (for like sever hyperkalemia or pulm edema).
- Delirium Tremens DT (or EtOH withdrawal needing too much Ativan per CIWA protocol; may need intubation & continuous sedation).
- Severe/ongoing GI bleeding w/ Hgb drop for close monitoring, blood transfusion & possible urgent GI scope (upper or lower).

Reconcile home meds
Thiss an important part of the management after MICU admission (or any hospital admission) & doing your 1st assessment/ work up along w/ initial Tx.
As a general role & due to the critical pt illness, constant ability to monitor the pt closely & the possibility of meds interactions; some meds should be held or switched to other forms.

Some examples:
- **Insulin drip** is preferred (stop PO diabetes meds in general in the hospital)
- **BP meds & diuretics** (hold in septic pts & carefully resume as BP tolerates)
- **Narcotics & pain meds** for chief complaint of AMS, HoTN or any complaints could be from the meds side effects. AMS is one of the signs of

organ dysfunction & it will be clouded w/ those meds on addition of possible HoTN & respiratory failure. Restart meds as appropriate when the diagnosis is clearer & pt is responding to Tx.

- **Psychiatric & sleep meds**: antipsychotic meds like Haldol (1st generation/better in cardiac disease), olanzapine/Quetiapine (2nd generation), & benzos (same reason for holding pain meds; resume as needed). Caution w/ benzos withdrawal seizures for chronic users.
- **Some meds w/ common side effects** like diphenhydramine (for itching; anticholinergic property causes AMS & urinary retention), Baclofen (for muscle spasm; causes AMS)
- **Hold meds which does NOT cause immediate benefits** like statins (if MICU admission is NOT from cardiac etiology), allopurinol, vitamins, etc (to ↓ meds interaction & ADR)

Shock

Shock is a state of ↓ tissue perfusion (mostly from HoTN), which can result in inadequate O_2 delivery for cellular needs (tissue ischemia). Tissues ischemia often results in organ dysfunction if severe or prolonged (usually >30 minutes).

Signs for shock: systolic BP <90, MAP<60, signs of end organ damage from hypoperfusion (↓ urine output, AMS, CP, lactic acidosis from the anaerobic metabolism) & lack of BP response after IV fluid challenge (usually after 2-3 Liters boluses).

Three main types of shock:
1. **Cardiogenic** (massive MI or pulm embolism),
2. **Septic** (from severe infx or anaphylaxis)
3. **Hypovolemic** (severe dehydration or bleeding).

Blood Pressure = Cardiac Output (Heart Rate x Stroke Volume) x Resistance

BP is consistent of few parameters including: peripheral resistance (mainly ↓ in septic shock), cardiac output (mainly ↓ in cardiogenic shock like in MI or CHF but also can be ↓ in septic shock du to the negative cardiac effect from the septic toxins) & preload or blood volume (mainly ↓ in bleeding/ dehydration & even in septic shock → hypovolemia occur due to ↑ capillary permeability & 3rd space loss).

In all types of shock, the therapeutic goals are to support tissues & organs that are dysfunctional or at risk of damage due to hypoperfusion & to restore perfusion if possible.

Perfusion can often be improved by administering some combination of intravenous fluids, vasopressors/ inotropic agents such as:

- **Norepinephrine (levophed):** which is strong α1 agonist (stronger than epinephrine) & β1 agonist (same as Epi)/ moderate β2 agonist (weaker than Epi). "Squeeze" good but **proarrhythmic due to β1 effect**.

> **Attention:** β2 agonist causes HoTN (receptors are in vessels) vs β1 agonist ↑ chronotropic and inotropic effect (receptors in the heart) vs α1 agonist in vessels (NOT in the heart) → vasoconstriction.

- **Phenylephrine:** which is strong α1 agonist. "Squeeze" good but do NOT affect the heart.
- **Vasopressin:** which is a V1 receptor agonist in the vascular smooth muscle of the vessels. Also "squeeze" w/o cardiac direct effect).
- **Dopamine & dobutamine:** less common
- **Epinephrine:** (β agonist mainly).

Understanding the cause of shock & reversing the cause of the abnormal physiologic parameter is the key to successful outcomes. Such directed Tx could include lysis of a massive pulm embolism causing cardiogenic shock or Tx of an infx causing septic shock. If ↑ fluid volume is likely to improve perfusion, intravenous fluids should be given liberally as boluses w/ immediate clinical reassessment (septic pts may need up to 6 liters in the 1st 6 hrs). The adoption of guidelines using physiologic parameters, such as central venous pressure, as targets for resuscitation has improved outcomes by encouraging more timely administration of needed fluids (mostly used is normal saline).

> **Attention**: the adaption of guidelines using physiologic parameters, such as central venous pressure CVP, as targets for resuscitation has improved outcomes by encouraging more timely administration of needed fluids (mostly used is Normal Saline).

Aggressive volume expansion is most important in pts w/ hypovolemic shock & has also been associated w/ improved outcomes in pts w/ septic shock. Concern about precipitating heart failure & pulm edema should NOT modify the need for large bolus volume administration (intubate if needed).

Sepsis
Sepsis is an exaggerated inflammatory response to an infectious stimulus & is characterized by a severe catabolic reaction, widespread endothelial dysfunction, & release of inflammatory agents. The mortality rate of pts w/ sepsis complicated by multiorgan failure may be greater than 70% to 90%; mortality rate can be estimated by adding 15% to 20% predicted mortality for each sepsis-induced organ dysfunction. The term/s:
- **Systemic inflammatory response syndrome (SIRS)** was introduced to describe findings of:
  1. Altered temperature (<36 or >38)
  2. Tachycardia (>100)

3. Hyperventilation (>20)
4. Abnormal WBC (<4, 000 or >12, 000) regardless of the cause (inflammatory or infectious).

- **Sepsis** is defined as SIRS plus suspected (or proven) infx (UTI, PNA, cellulitis etc).
- **Severe sepsis** is associated w/ systemic effects including: HoTN, ↓ urine output, or metabolic acidosis.
- **Septic shock** is sepsis w/ persistent organ hypoperfusion despite adequate initial fluid resuscitation, which is usually 30cc/kg (like 3 liters for 100kg pt. That requires vasopressor agents to maintain blood pressure).

Attention: No septic shock w/o persistant HoTN (NOT responding to IV fluid) but sepsis can happen even w/o HoTN.

Management
Treat infx (empiric abx like vanc/zosyn w/ in 30 minutes of recognizing sepsis, if possible) & optimize tissue perfusion (by aggressive fluid resuscitation & vasopressors). Repetitive fluid challenges are performed by giving a 500 to 1000 mL bolus of crystalloid over short intervals while assessing response to target central venous pressure (normal is 8-10, higher number is may be better in case of septic shock).

Most pts need 4 to 6 L of fluid in the first 6 hrs, & a frequent error is underestimating the intravascular volume deficit & the amount of fluid required. Use of crystalloid or colloid is likely equivalent. Vasopressor therapy should be started immediately if the initial fluid challenge fails to restore adequate blood pressure & organ perfusion.

Prolonged hypoperfusion results in worsening ischemia & organ failure. Vasopressor therapy w/ norepinephrine, vasopressin, or phenylephrine is frequently needed to restore perfusion during life-threatening HoTN.

No trials have established a single superior vasopressor agent. Norepinephrine, vasopressor, phenylephrine are 1st-line agents for correcting HoTN in septic shock. Vasopressor agents can be used concurrently w/ fluid resuscitation in life-threatening HoTN.

Being at the upper side of fluid resuscitation is better than under resuscitation & intubate prn if pulm edema & CHF is a concern. Get lactic acid q4-6hrs & monitor the trend; down trending is reassuring & up trending may indicate plan/intervention changing.

Pain, delirium, & sedation in the ICU

- **For pain:** pts in the ICU may NOT be sufficiently interactive to give valid responses. Physiological indicators such as hypertension & tachycardia correlate poorly w/ more intuitively valid measures of pain, but pain scales such as **Critical Care Pain Observation Tool (available online)** which consider facial expression, body movement, vent compliance (for intubated pts) & muscle tension to provide structured & repeatable assessments & it is currently the best available methods for assessing pain. **Tx:** fentanyl IV drip, patches or boluses/morphine IV.
- **For sedation:** it is widely used in the ICU & mostly for intubation. In general, no sedative drug is clearly superior to all others. Sedatives that are commonly used in the ICU: benzodiazepines (GABA agonist) likeVerced (midazolam) & ativan (lorazepam) vs short-acting intravenous (short-acting & titratable drugs) anesthetic agent propofol, & Precedex (dexmedetomidine; α2-

adrenoceptor agonist). Each one has certain benefit & quality. **Precedex have advantages over benzodiazepines**, since it produces analgesia, causes less respiratory depression, & seemingly provides a qualitatively different type of sedation in which patients are more interactive & so potentially better able to communicate their needs (& the best to extubate on if sedation is needed).

- **For delirium:** Delirium is a nonspecific but generally reversible manifestation of acute illness that appears to have many causes, including recovery from a sedated or oversedated state. The pathophysiology of delirium that is associated w/ critical illness remains largely uncharacterized & may vary depending on the cause. Duration of delirium was significantly ↓ w/ early mobilization & interruptions in sedation. **Prevent** w/ Olanzapine (2nd G antipsychotics) & **treat** w/ haldol PO/IV or quetiapine PO (even Precedex drip can be used in hyperactive delirium & showed superiority in some studies over benzos & haldol). Diagnosis of delirium is associated w/ ↑ mortality (estimated as a 10% ↑ in the relative risk of death for each day of delirium). Sedation w/ Precedex rather than benzos appears to reduce the incidence of delirium in the ICU.

Special considerations
- **Assess the need for lines** such as arterial line, central line, hemodialysis line, foley cath.

Attention: short line (like peripheral large lines) are better for resuscitation than long/ narrow lines (like PICC/ central lines) due to ↑ fluid flow resistance with ↑ line length and ↓ line radius.

- **Consider prophylactic meds** like GI ulcers w/ PPI & DVT w/ heparin SQ & check for decubitus ulcers in all ICU pts.
- **Low-dose corticosteroids** as indicated in septic shock refractory to fluids & vasopressor therapy
- **Critically ill pts w/ anemia** who are NOT bleeding & who do NOT have acute coronary syndrome appear to do better w/ more conservative threshold for blood transfusion (Hgb level ≤7 g/dL [70 g/L]) for blood transfusion).
- **Bicarbonate should NOT be used** for the purpose of improving hemodynamics or reducing vasopressor requirement when treating lactic acidosis w/ a pH higher than 7.15.
- **Always consider:** avoiding malnutrition, employing therapist-driven weaning protocols, using sedation protocols w/ a daily interruption in ventilated pts, using intermittent or bolus sedation rather than continuous infusions, & avoiding neuromuscular blockade as possible.
- **Unconscious adult pts w/ spontaneous circulation after out-of-hospital cardiac arrest should be cooled** to 32°C to 34°C for 12 to 24 hrs when the initial rhythm was VF. Such cooling may also be beneficial for other rhythms or in-hospital cardiac arrest. Usually prognosis is poor for pts whom did NOT gain meaningful communication in the next 48-72 hrs (it is better to wait to tell the prognosis to the family until that time pass)
- **Glasgow Coma Scale (GCS)** is a neurological scale that aims to give a reliable, objective way of recording the conscious state of a person for initial as well as subsequent assessment (**available online**).

> **Attention:** assessing mental status (like s/p code or coma from trauma) should be done "off sedation" which could be needed for intubation or seizure control. No meaningful communication after 3days from the coma (off sedation) has poor prognosis.

- **Sedation holiday** involves stopping the sedative infusions & allowing the patient to be awake. The infusion should only be restarted once the patient is fully awake & obeying commands or until they became uncomfortable or agitated & deemed to require the resumption of sedation. Ideally, this should be performed on a daily basis. This strategy has been shown to ↓ the duration of mechanical ventilation, length of stay in ICU, & ICU delirium w/o increasing adverse events such as self-extubation.
- **Code blue:** ACLS algorithm (**available online**). **As a quick review:**
  1. Unresponsive?
  2. Pulseless?
  3. Start chest compression
  4. IV access/heart rhythm? (place monitor pads) /intubation?
  5. Conisder Elictrical cardioversion (V fib/tach/SVT?), IV meds (epi/HCO3/Mag/IV fluid/amio) prn
  6. Send for basic blood work (CBG, CBC, CMP, lactate, troponin, D Dimer, ABG, etc)
  7. Check the chart, nurse, or primary team for any possible etiology, recent meds or intervention could be related to the code (like high insulin dose or new meds).
  Assess pulse & heart rhythm q2min → check BP if you had *Return Of Spontaneous Circulation* (*ROSC*) & transfer to ICU. Attempt to call family to update them. **Do not do chest compression on an "awake person".**

2. Acute respiratory failure & basics for oxygen therapy

Respiratory failure results from either hypoxia (low O_2) or hypercapnia (elevated CO_2), or both.

Hypoxemic respiratory failure etiology:

- **Diffusion defect:** ↓ diffusion capacity for any reason like pulm edema & ARDS, **measured by:**
  1. PaO_2 (artrial)/FiO_2 (alveolar) ratio: normal ratio is >500 which is the result of 100 mm Hg dissolved O2 / 21% air O2. The lower the ratio →the worse the defect (the shunt). In severe ARDS the ratio is <100.
  2. A-a gradiet: normal is 4-10 (depends on age too). The higher the gradient → the worse the defect (calculator is **available online** for the two previous ratio & gradient).
- **Hypoventilation:** ↓ minute ventilation leads to ↑ $PaCO_2$ & ↓ PaO_2. **Etiology:** CNS depression, Obesity Hypoventilation syndrome OHS (Pickwickian syndrome), Obstructive Sleep Apenia OSA or Narcotics overdose.
- **Hypovolemia, poor cardiac output, MI**
- **V/Q mismatch:** pulm embolism, Pulm HTN, COPD, Asthma, ILD. Corrects w/ supplemental O_2
- **Shunt:** perfusion to non-ventilated alveoli (collapsed or flooded with fluid, pus or blood) or communication w/ arterial/venous system. From ARDS, PNA, AVM, congenital heart disease, PFO w/ right to left flow. **This does NOT correct w/ supplemental O_2.** Rather, hypoxia is reversed w/ Positive End Expiratory Pressure PEEP support to "recruits" & "open" affected alveoli.
- ↓ **FiO_2 or ↓ total O_2** →O_2 replaced by other gases or ↓ O_2 from high altitude

Hypercapnic respiratory failure etiology:

- **CNS disorders/$\downarrow$ ventilator drive/drug overdose, OSA**
- **Peripheral nerve disorders:** Guillan Barre Syndrome, ALS, West Nile Virus, ICU acquired myopathy/paresis
- **NMJ disorders:** Myasthenia Gravis, Botulism
- **Muscle disorders:** Muscular Dystrophy
- **Lung:** obstructive lung disease (COPD, Asthma, & CF)
- **Chest wall disorders:** obesity, chest trauma

O_2 facts

- Room Air RA has 21% O_2 (FiO$_2$ is 21%)
- Supplemental O_2 can $\uparrow$ FiO$_2$ to 100% (depends on the delivery method)
- 97% O_2 transported to tissues bound to Hgb, 3% dissolved in plasma
- ABG measures PaO$_2$: pressure of O_2 dissolved in plasma (80-100mmHg is normal)
- O_2 saturation can be measured via pulse ox; normal value >94% (NOT very accurate as it is affected by peripheral perfusion & does NOT tell the CO_2 status, get ABG for better assessment)
- 1L of supplemental O_2 will $\uparrow$ FiO$_2$ ~3% (like 3L O_2 in facemask will $\uparrow$ FiO$_2$ to 30%, 21% room air+9%=30%)

Methods of oxygen delivery

- **Nasal Cannula:** can deliver1-6 L/min; FiO$_2$ 24-40%
- **Simple Face Mask:** can deliver5-10 L/min; FiO$_2$ 30-60%. Indicated if pt requires higher O_2 concentration; flow rate can be adjusted as well to prevent re-breathing of exhaled CO_2
- **Non-rebreather mask:** can deliver10-15L/min; FiO$_2$ 60-80%. It has a one way valve which allows exhaled CO_2 to leave mask; $\downarrow$ CO_2

- ↑ **flow device:** Delivers O_2 at rates above normal inspiratory flow rate, maintains fixed FiO_2
- **Venturi mask:** can deliver4-12 L/min; FiO_2 24-50%. Uses a nozzle to ↑ O_2 flow & mix w/ air
- **Aerosol devices:** Produce fine mist that can be delivered w/ face mask, tracheostomy (trach) collar or T piece (commonly used before considering extubation to assess spontaneous breathing as it is NOT connected on the ventilator)

Ventilator basics

Non-invasive positive pressure ventilation (NIPPV) , sometimes called "NIV", consists of delivery of positive airway pressure breaths w/o the use of an endotracheal tube or tracheostomy. In general, the interface between the critically ill pt & NPPV device is a tight-fitting mask. It ↓ the work of breathing & results in less energy expenditure to support a pt's required minute ventilation. It is the standard of care for managing moderate to severe COPD exacerbations (to prevent intubation).

Other indications: Cardiogenic pulm edema (treat the edema mechanically until the diuresis work), post-extubation, immune compromised pts (due to ↑ risk for nosocomial infx like intubation associated PNA) & other pts w/ hypoxemic respiratory failure.

> **Attention:** NIV, Non-rebreather & intubation (w/ ↑ RR) are maybe the best interventions to ↓ CO_2.

Contraindications: Severe acidemia, inability to protect airway (in case of vomiting), AMS, aspiration risk, upper GI bleed, impending cardiac/respiratory arrest & Uncooperative pt requiring sedation.

> **Attention**: Non-invasive positive pressure ventilation has the potential to worsen outcomes by excessively delaying, rather than preventing, intubation in high-risk populations. Elective intubation is appropriate for pts w/ acute respiratory failure who do NOT respond to a 1- to 2-hr trial of non-invasive support.

Invasive Mechanical Ventilation: indicated for airway protection & acute respiratory failure, inability to tolerate NIV for above listed contraindications. Modes:
1. **Assist control:** preset tidal volume or pressure. 1st choice in most clinical situations, used commonly for ARDS.
2. **Synchronized Intermittent Mandatory Ventilation SIMV:** delivers preset TV, minimum RR. Spontaneous breathes above minimum mandatory RR triggers variable tidal volume. Spontaneous breaths & mandatory breaths are synchronized to reduce breath stacking/air trapping.
3. **Pressure Support:** Inspiratory pressure support to ↓ work of breathing. Close monitoring required; dependent on pt's lung mechanics.

Weaning
Is the process by which a pt is liberated from mechanical ventilation. Pts are candidates for weaning when they are hemodynamically stable & have recovered from respiratory failure. They should have a cough that is strong enough to clear secretions, a ↓ secretion burden, & a patent upper airway. The rapid shallow breathing index (RSBI) is a method to test the readiness of a pt for weaning & should be measured daily. It is defined as the ratio of the respiratory rate to tidal volume (f/VT). If the f/VT is greater than 105, there is a 95% chance that a spontaneous breathing trial will be unsuccessful; if it is less than 105, there is an 80% chance of success.

Spontaneous breathing trials are usually done by placing the pt on a T-piece where no positive pressure is delivered (only supplemental O_2) or by adjusting the ventilator so that it applies only enough pressure to overcome the resistance of the endotracheal tube. Weaning parameters can be done by Respiratory Therapist (RT) when pt on T-piece →suggest extubation if parameters are good (numbers are **available online**). **Clinically:** if pt is tolerating T-piece for >1 hour once or twice w/o distress like tachycardia & tachypnea (& the original etiology is improving like pulmonary edema or PNA) ± ABG is good →extubate

Daily interruption of sedation (sedation holidays) & spontaneous breathing trials should be used as a standard of care for appropriate pts in critical care units. Their use will shorten the need for mechanical ventilation by an average of 1.5 days, dramatically ↓ the number of pts who require mechanical ventilation for more than 3 weeks, ↓ ICU length of stay, & lower 1-year mortality. Direct extubation to NPPV is effective at weaning pts w/ obstructive lung disease from mechanical ventilation.

Special considerations

- **Positive end-expiratory pressure** is the 1st-line approach to correcting shunt-associated hypoxemia in pts w/ acute respiratory distress syndrome, but it is less applicable in the setting of focal disease.
- **In the intensive care unit:** daily interruption of sedation & spontaneous breathing trials lead to more rapid extubation & lower rate of mechanical ventilation
- **Ventilator-associated PNA** can be prevented by the routine use of protocols that require elevating the head of the bed by 30 degrees & hastening time to extubation.
- **Lung Volumes:** RV: residual volume in lungs at maximal expiration. ERV: air exhaled after normal expiration. TV: air that enters/exits lungs during normal respiration ~500cc. FRC: functional

reserve: RV+ERV. Total Lung Capacity TLC: RV+ERV+TV+ IRV

- **Vent Settings:**
  Minute ventilation MV = respiratory rate RR x Tidal volume TV. **RR** usually 12
  FiO$_2$: start w/ 100% FiO$_2$, then titrate down to goal PaO$_2$ ≥ 60mmHg (or O$_2$ sat >92%).
  PEEP: 5 cm H20 is commonly used; high levels used in ARDS & cardiogenic pulm edema to improve oxygenation. ↓**TV** (6mL/kg) → ↓ mortality in ARDS.
- **Atelectasis** is an important cause of hypoxemia in surgical (preventable by early use of incentive spirometry before & after surgery) & mechanically ventilated pts.
- The need for large amounts of supplemental O$_2$ in pts w/ exacerbations of COPD or asthma should prompt consideration of **alternative diagnoses** (as those diagnosis, usually, easily corrected w/ increasing FiO$_2$)
- **A slightly elevated, or even normal, arterial PCO$_2$** in a pt w/ an asthma exacerbation may indicate impending respiratory arrest (consider intubation). Pts w/ a severe asthma exacerbation that does NOT respond to 1 hr of aggressive bronchodilator therapy are candidates for admission to the intensive care unit.
- **Pts w/ acute upper airway obstruction (like in angioedema) should be closely monitored** & low threshold for intubation should be considered given the difficulty of endotracheal tube placement in this population. Consider ENT consult for laryngeal scope & MICU evaluation for Angioedema pts (pt on lisinopril w/ lips/tongue sudden swelling/hoarseness) even if they do NOT look in respiratory distress at the time of presentation due to the high risk of sudden deterioration.
- **The physiologic hallmark of ARDS is acute (<1week) hypoxemia:** (w/ bilateral infiltration w/o

other lung pathology like nodules/pleural effusion or cardiac pulm edema), which is typically corrected w/ mechanical ventilation combined w/ supplemental O_2 & positive end-expiratory pressure. In pts w/ ARDS, limiting tidal volumes, minimizing plateau pressure, optimizing positive end-expiratory pressure, & reducing FIO_2 to less than 0.6 may help prevent ventilator-associated lung injury. Usually ARDS recovery/Tx is long (if pt recovers in 2-3 days →not ARDS)

- **Hypercapnic:** is tolerated much better than hypoxia
- "**Trach collar**" is a term to describe pts who had tracheostomy & on ventilator (for maybe pressure support)
- "**Weaning on sedation**": is maybe useful for anxious pts, especially if the parameters & ABG is good on T-piece trials (anxiety from feeling thy can NOT breathe independently from maybe long mechanical ventilation).

3. IV lines, IV fluids, Foley catheters & contrast material

IV lines: Most of the hospital pts need peripheral IV lines for IV meds, blood draws, fluids, blood, or resuscitation in case of dehydration or bleeding (sometimes you need 2 large bore peripheral IV lines for faster fluid resuscitation).

Central lines (intra-jugular & peripherally inserted central cath PICC) are indicated for the following: long-term hospitalization (blood withdrAwal), delivery of certain meds maybe NOT appropriate peripherally (e.g. 20 meq K or >D5% fluid), critical pts w/ HoTN & needing vasopressors, small peripheral veins or "hard stick", & long term IV therapy (e.g., infective endocarditis requiring IV abx for 6 weeks).

> **Attention:** Be cautious w/ HD pts as they may need any possible dialysis port access & any central IV access should be done per nephrology recommendations (except in emergencies).

Fluids: Most commonly used are Normal Saline (NS), Dextrose 5% water (D5W), D5 NS, D5 1/2NS.

Fluid replacement: In cases of fluid deficits, which can manifest w/ HoTN or tachycardia due to bleeding (internal or external), dehydration (sweating, excessive diuresis, diarrhea, etc), & septic shock (no frank fluid deficits & it is more of ↓ vessels resistance).
The rate of correction of volume depletion depends upon severity. For pts w/ severe volume depletion or hypovolemic shock, we recommend administration of 1 to 2 liters of isotonic saline as rapidly as possible (~999cc/hr) in an attempt to restore tissue perfusion. Fluid repletion is continued at a rapid rate until the

clinical signs of hypovolemia improve (eg, ↓ blood pressure, tachycardia, ↓ urine output, impaired mental status or up trending of lactic acid).
For pts w/ CHF you can do 250cc or 500cc boluses & evaluate for pulm edema in between by assessing SOB & breath sounds (intubate as needed).

Maintenance fluid: In cases of NPO status, where pt canNOT tolerate PO intake for any reason (eg, pancreatitis, gastroenteritis). Usually it is 75-100ml/h & total of 2 L/day (which is going to be equal to the insensible water loss in sweat, metabolism, & stool, as well as minimal urinary output). This rate, however, is NOT sufficient for replacing any fluid deficits/hypovolemia/dehydration & it is usually after to replace the deficits aggressively as above.

Special consideration:
- **Free water flushes (through NG tube)** can be considered for Tx of hypernatremia. Giving fluids through the GI system is preferred over IV unless it is urgent.
- **Reassess the need for IV fluids on a daily bases** to prevent iatrogenic pulm edema especially for pts w/ CHF (systolic or diastolic/preserved EF). Euvolemic pts who are tolerating PO intake do NOT need IV fluids.
- **Be aware of dilutional anemia** (↓ in RBC, WBC & platelets).
- **HoTN refractory** to the initial 2-3 L fluids resuscitation may indicate the need for MICU transfer & BP support meds (epinephrine/phenylephrine/vasopressin/norepinephrine). In general, the need for 3 or more BP support meds indicates very poor prognosis. HoTN refractory to fluid resuscitation differentiates sepsis (HoTN respond to IV fluid & no need for vasopressors) from septic shock (persistent HoTN despite IV fluid & need Vasopressors).

- **Some conditions require a lot of fluid resuscitation** (>4-6L of NS in the first 6 hrs), such as DKA, HHNS, pancreatitis, severe dehydration, & septic shock.

Foley catheter: ↑ the risk of UTI & needs daily assessments in deciding to whether to continue or to discontinue. It is indicated for urinary retention (like BPH) & strict ins/outs monitoring, especially when assessing a CHF pt's response to diuresis or assessing a shock pt's response to fluid resuscitation (consider a condom cath for cooperative men w/ no obstruction/still ↑ UTI risk to 2folds).
Other pts requiring intake/output monitoring include: critically ill pts, perioperative pts, & end-of-life pts needing palliative care.
Bladder scans (better) or in/out Foley cath can differentiate between urinary retention & anuria (no urine in the bladder like in AKI). Consider a Foley cath in place if the scan shows >350-400cc post voidal residual urine (means urinary retention).
Urine culture from indwelling foley cath may NOT be accurate due to colonization (which does NOT indicate abx use).

Contrast material (IV): CT (Iodine based) or MRI (Gadolinium) w/ IV contrast is useful when you are looking for infx or cancer. Contrast induced nephropathy can occur w/ already damaged kidney (CKD at any stage). If IV contrast is essential in a pt w/ mildly elevated Cr, you can use Acetylcysteine (both prior & post-study) & aggressive IV hydration (NS 200-250 cc/hr) prior to contrast administration.

Special consideration:
- **Gadolinium should be avoided in ESRD** even if on HD due to the risk of nephrogenic systemic fibrosis (NSF), thickening of the skin & other organs.
- **Barium contrast (NOT water soluble)** administered PO or rectally along w/ X-ray or CT can evaluate for

GI pathology. Gastrografin (water soluble) should be used as contrast material if you suspect perforated esophagus.

- **Cardiac catheterization w/ IV contrast** is a common procedure. Kidney function should be monitored before & after the procedure (usually in the next 24 hrs) for AKI ($\uparrow$ in Cr >30% of the baseline).

- **Try to avoid using two IV contrast studies** w/ in 24 hours period, like left heart cath & CTA (especially in case of kidney disease). Consider MRI as a second study if CT w/ contrast was done earlier at the same day (if possible).

4. Chest pain (CP)

An internist should be able to promptly recognize CP, form a differential diagnosis, & be able to treat accordingly. Remember, the most important part of your assessment is obtaining complete pt hx.

History & physical exam
- **Onset**
- **Location**
- **Duration:** just happened few hours ago vs constant for 1 month (later is somewhat reassuring as pt can not have cardiac/ischemic pain for 1 month).
- **Characteristics**: Sharp? Achy? Dull? Crushing?
- **Aggravating factors** that trigger or worsen the CP
- **Relieving factors**/trial to relieve pain (e.g. whether Tylenol or NTG relieves the pain)
- **Radiation**: such as to the shoulder, back, jaw, or abdomen.
- **Timing of CP**: Does the pain wake the pt from sleep? Does the pain occur at rest or when working in the backyard? Similarity to or difference from pain during previous MI (alarming if it is similar to the last MI).
- **Severity:** (1-10 scale), ever went to zero (w/ like Tylenol or NTG)?

Others: Associated Sx (N/V, diaphoresis, cough, dyspnea, fever, edema, abdominal pain), family hx of cardiac disease or other causes of CP, meds (e.g. ASA, β-blocker, NTG). Also, obtain all cardiac hx such as CHF Sx, chronic angina, smoking, any hx of cardiac intervention or diagnostic tests such as stress testing or cardiac catheterization (including coronary anatomy).

CV	Aortic dissection	Sudden onset of tearing/ripping CP that usually radiates to the back, & may present w/ hemodynamic instability, such as HoTN & tachycardia. Type A affects the ascending aorta (surgical case) while Type B affects the descending aorta (medical case). Control HTN aggressively.
	Acute Coronary Syndrome	Typically ischemic pain is crushing, substernal & left sided CP ("elephant on chest"), which can radiate to the jaw or down the left arm. Associated Sx: diaphoresis, SOB & N/V. If EKG shows ischemic changes or troponin is positive → NSTEMI or STEMI. If EKG shows ischemic changes & troponin is negative → unstable angina (usually >15 minutes). Remember, women & diabetics can present w/ vague non-specific Sx like N/V, so you must be careful in ruling out ACS. If stable angina→ usually lasts 1-5 minutes/ brought on by exertion & or emotion/ relieved by rest or NTG.
	Pericarditis	Friction rub on auscultation, pleuritic CP, EKG shows diffuse ST elevation (down concave) in most of the leads (but ST depression in aVR) & diffuse PR segment depression, pain improves w/ leaning forward (or sometimes just w/ positional changes).
	Arrhythmia	Order an EKG whenever someone presents w/ CP (also consider telemetry).
	Myocarditis	Fever w/ cardiac/CHF Sx. Cardiac arrhythmias is common.

Pulm	PE	Acute onset of dyspnea, tachycardia, & tachypnea w/ pleuritic CP (usually w/ pts have risk factors like immobilization).
	PNA	Pleuritic CP that worsens w/ deep inspiration or cough; can be associated w/ fever, cough, dyspnea, & tachypnea. Dull to percussion & crackles on auscultation.
	PTX	Usually sudden onset of dyspnea/tachypnea, ↓or absent breath sounds on the affected side.
GI	GERD	Usually postprandial, w/ a burning, gnawing pain, which worsens w/ recumbency. It can mimic cardiac CP (try PPI after ruling out cardiac cause for those w/ cardiac risk factors).
	PUD	Sharp abdominal pain, that radiates from abdomen to chest
Others	**Esoph-ageal spasm**	Severe pain w/ eating can be relieved by nitroglycerin. Therefore, it can be difficult to differentiate cardiac origin from esophagus spasm. Tx: CCB
	Costo-chondritis	Reproducible by palpating the affected area or during chest movement. Pinpoint CP is unlikely to be cardiac.
	Anxiety	Can be similar to cardiac CP in that it can present w/ crushing CP w/ tachycardia, diaphoresis & is brought on by emotional stress.
	HZV (shingles)	Presents w/ a classic rash w/ in a single dermatome. Though during early stages of disease, rash & vesicles may be absent but pt may complain of severe pain in the dermatomal distribution.

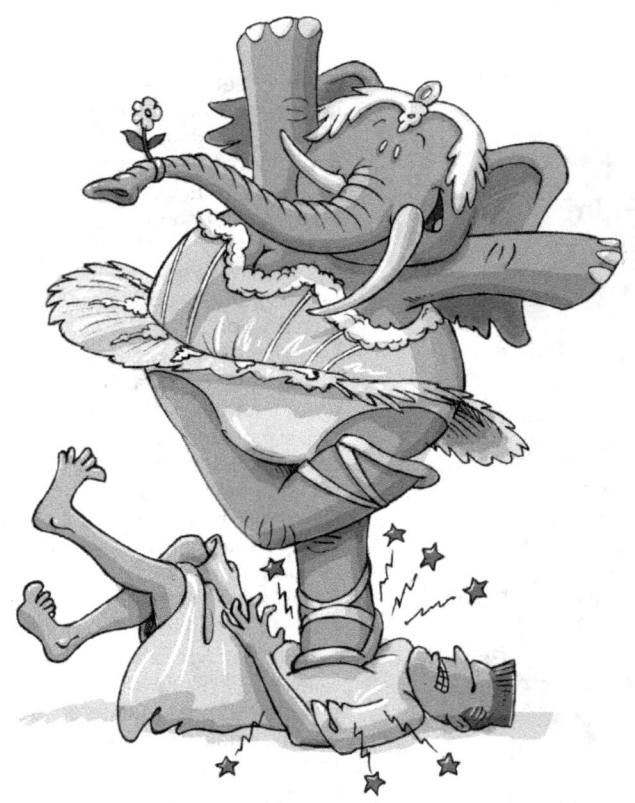

Chest heaviness is typical for acute coronary syndrome.

Management

- Vital signs (ACLS for unstable pt), EKG (compare to prior EKGs if available) & ask above questions (considering the DDx in the above table).
- **If pain appears cardiac in origin,** give ASA 325mg (± Plavix), NTG SL, β-blocker (metoprolol or carvedilol), & Heparin. High dose statins (80mg atorvastatin) are indicated in 24 hours, as well as ACEi like lisinopril in also 24hours as clinical trials

support mortality benefits (NOT in ACS guidelines but recommended).

- Avoid NTG for inferior wall MI because the heart is preload/volume dependent. Also, avoid β blocker if pt is bradycardic (<60). Dual antiplatelet therapy (ASA +Plavix) ↓ mortality especially with loading dose of Plavix (300 0r 600 mg) followed by maintenance dose (75mg).
- Plavix usually delay CABG surgery (or any elective surgery) 5 days due to high bleeding risk until the medicine "wash out" from the body.
- Rule/Out MI or "ROMI" is a common hospital admission for pts w/ CP presented to the emergency department & they did NOT have cardiac enzymes elevation & ischemic EKG changes; regardless of the CP quality (typical or NOT typical for MI). Cardiac enzymes (troponin I) x 3 Q6 hrs is needed for those pts to note the trend (you can also repeat EKGs Q15-30 minutes PRN especially if CP recurs). NSTEMI is diagnosed when troponin is elevated after the chest pain.

> **Attention:** Troponin elevation can happen in some cases, which is NOT related to coronary occlusion like kidney injury (acute or chronic), tachycardia (for any reason like a fib), HTN/HoTN, and infx/sepsis.

- If the troponins continue to show an upward trend, you need to continue trending it until they begin decreasing or at least plateau status.
- Call STEMI code or cardiology "stat" for any chest pain with ST elevation or any other equivalent (poor q wave progression or new LBBB)
- If there are EKG changes, elevated troponin levels, ongoing CP or unstable vitals → call Cardiology. Start the pt on heparin drip w/ a

loading dose protocol, assuming there is no contraindication (weight dose Lovenox is also an alternative to heparin drip, if the kidney function is normal).

Common EKG Changes Seen in STEMI

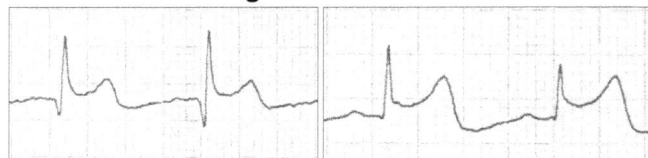

- MONA (morphine, O_2, NTG, ASA) for ACS treatment is outdated & incorrect. O_2 did NOT show benefit unless pt is hypoxic. Morphine may sedate & conceal ongoing ischemia; use morphine w/ caution for chest pain (after NTG sublingual or IV drip for ongoing chest pain). Always use ASA & NTG if NOT contraindicated.
- If pain appears GI in origin, consider PPI or GI cocktail (antacid + Donnatal + lidocaine).
- Always consider the possibility of a PE, pneumothorax, or aortic dissection, as they need very high suspicion.
- If pulm embolism is high on the differential →order EKG (sinus tachycardia), ABG (hypoxia & possible hypocapnia from tachypnea), & chest CTA. Treat w/ heparin drip or lovenox (if NOT contraindicated). If a pulm embolism is somewhat likely, you can obtain a D-dimer assay (low specificity but high sensitivity); discouraged for in pt setting due to low specificity. Consider lower extremity venous US if you suspect DVT & treat w/ heparin/warfarin (or any anticoagx meds) if positive (same Tx as for pulm embolism & hence may NOT need CTA w/o chest pain).
- If PNA is high on the differential, order a CXR, blood/sputum cultures & empiric abx, if appropriate.

- If aortic dissection is high on the differential, obtain a CXR (if hemodynamically stable) to check for mediastinal widening, & consider CTA along w/ vascular surgery consultation as soon as possible.

5. Shortness of breath (SOB)

The subjective sensation of breathlessness commonly referred to as dyspnea.

History
- Is this SOB acute (pulm embolism or PNA), chronic (COPD/CHF), or acute on chronic (COPD/CHF exacerbation)?
- On rest (possible ACS or severe CHF) or exertion (typical for CHF); ask about the baseline SOB, if any, & how worse it is now (how many blocks or feet can they walk?)
- Associated Sx such as cough/sputum (PNA), CP (ACS, PNA), palpitations (a fib or any arrhythmias), fever (PNA), orthopnea/ paroxysmal nocturnal dyspnea PND/ peripheral edema (CHF), legs swelling or weight gain.
- New events or meds near the onset including trauma, IV fluids (pulm edema). Assess adherence to meds.
- Urine output (low in oliguric AKI & severe CHF)

Physical exam
- **Vital signs:** including O_2 sat.
- **Lungs**: respiratory distress, non-labored respirations, accessory muscle use, midline trachea, crackles, wheezes, stridor, egophony, symmetry of breath sounds
- **Cardiac**: JVD (most sensitive/specific sign for CHF), carotids, rate/rhythm, murmurs or rubs, loud P2 (pulm HTN), RV heave (due to RV dilation) & S3.
- **Neuro**: mental status, confused, drowsy (gives an idea of cerebral O_2 delivery)
- **Extremities**: edema, cool vs. warm, capillary refill, & cyanosis (peripheral vs. central)

Work-up

- CXR (check: PNA/COPD)
- EKG (check arrhythmias/sinus tachycardia in pulm embolus/ pulm edema in CHF/ cardiac ischemia)
- ABG (hypoxia in pulm embolus, pulm edema, COPD exacerbation & PNA)
- CBC (Hgb for symptomatic anemia & WBC for PNA)
- BMP (check for AKI)
- BNP (check for CHF exacerbation); >100 is abnormal (>50 for obese pts, unknown why but it is like BNP dissolve in fat).
- Troponin (check for ACS).
- Consider CT angiogram if strong suspicion of pulm embolism (If unable to obtain CT w/ contrast because of kidney injury, obtain a V/Q scan)

Differential diagnosis

- **Pneumonia PNA:** diagnosed clinically. CXR opacities is suggestive (dehydration can delay opacities. If high suspicion, hydrate & repeat CXR), chest CT scan is more sensitive for PNA & can be ordered in complicated picture (very sick pt w/o clear clinical PNA, differentiate between CHF vs PNA vs pulm embolism). Calculate CURB-65 or PNA severity index (estimates mortality, & helps decide where the pt should be treated: in pt, out pt, or ICU).
  CURB-65: all are given 1 point for being present. If pt receives 2 or more points, consider in pt Tx vs out pt; w/ close follow up. If they receive4-5, consider ICU care (online calculator is available & can give estimated mortality rates)
  - **C**onfusion
  - **BUN** > 19 mg/dL
  - **R**espiratory Rate > 30
  - **B**P: Systolic < 90 mmHg or Diastolic < 60 mmHg

- o Age >**65**
- **CHF:** exacerbation (findings: BNP>100/possible pulm edema on x-ray/peripheral edema on exam)
- **MI/ischemia:** dyspnea on rest or exertion can be an angina equivalent (usually SOB is from CHF or lung issues & CP is from ischemia but they overlap).
- **Pulmonary embolism (PE):** common etiology for acute SOB, often difficult to rule in/out by hx/exam. Consider if pt has risk factors; calculate the Wells' Criteria score (online calculator is available). Treat w/ heparin drip/lovenox before waiting for the CTA results (if NOT contraindicated).

> **Attention:** D Dimer testing is discouraged for in pt setting (especially if admitted >2days) due to false positive results.
> In the ED or out pt: Consider D Dimer for low to moderate PE suspicion accordning to Wells's criteria & directly go to CTA for high suspicion (after starting heparin).

- **Pleural effusion:** from CHF vs. Malignancy vs. Infx (x-ray & BNP can be very informative)
- **Volume overload:** from various reasons like CHF or iatrogenic from excessive IV fluid. JVD & LE edema is suggestive & CXR may show pulmonary congestion or frank pulm edema. BNP may be elevated. Stop fluid & diurese (repeat CXR prn to follow resolution).
- **Arrhythmia**: can cause SOB even w/o CHF/ischemia
- **Anemia or anxiety.**
- **Aspiration PNA:** common in pts w/ altered mental status (needs time to show on CXR)
- **Bronchospasm:** can occur in CHF, PNA, & asthma/COPD (trial of jet neb w/ albuterol can help diagnose & treat).

- **Upper airway obstruction:** often acute onset, stridor/focal wheezing (call for ENT evaluation)
- **ARDS:** usually in hospitalized pts & most likely in the ICU (PaO_2 /FiO_2 usually <100)
- **TRALI (Transfusion related acute lung injury):** Usually very rapid onset post-transfusion (usually NOT more than 24 hrs)
- **Pneumothorax:** acute onset, pleuritic CP, consider in intubated pts (especially if peak & plateau pressures are elevated) or post procedures like thoracentesis.
- **Cardiac tamponade:** consider when pt has signs of isolated right heart failure; look for Beck's Triad of Sx ($\downarrow$ BP, distended neck veins, & distant, muffled heart sounds). Check pulsus paradoxus & obtain EKG (should see sinus tachycardia; can see electrical alternans & $\downarrow$ voltage), along w/ the CXR done routinely w/ SOB (if it is large enough you will see a "globular" or enlarged cardiac silhouette on CXR). Have a higher suspicion for this in your dialysis pts, as well as post-cath pts.
- **Others:**
  - **Sepsis**
  - **Metabolic acidosis** (cause tachypnea to blow off CO_2 & compensate)
  - **Massive ascites**
  - **Anaphylaxis** reactions from meds/others (should see signs of edema, urticaria, HoTN); **Tx:** with epinephrine (most important), hydrocortisone, Benadryl, & Famotidine.
  - **Narcotic overdose** can cause respiratory depression, which may NOT manifest as frank SOB feeling due to hypoventilation (give naloxone IV).

Management
1. **Oxygen:** Goal is a PaO_2 > 60 (need ABG), or O_2 sat > 90%. Nasal cannula delivers max FiO_2 ~35-40%, then switch to Venturi mask (delivers up to 50%),

NIPPV (CCU/MICU admission is warranted once pt needed NIPPV; indicate a sick pt needing intensive care). Respiratory Therapist can help w/ nebulizers, suction, masks, ABGs, PO/nasal airways.

2. **Bronchodilator** (Albuterol): Pts w/ wheezing from any etiology can benefit from bronchodilators. All that wheezes is NOT always asthma (e.g. CHF, PNA). Nebulizer: albuterol +/- ipratropium for your COPD & Asthma pts .Use Xopenex for wheezing w/ arterial fibrillation (less β1 agonist effect; less cardiac effect/tachycardia). **In asthma exacerbation:** check peak flows (on PFT) & obtain Gram stain & culture of the sputum.

3. **Lasix**: on pts w/ hx or exam consistent with CHF. Monitor Serum Cr, & be careful w/ CKD pts (they may need higher Lasix doses to diurese). **Diuresis:** double the home dose of Lasix (or any other & give it IV. You can ↑ the dose later if there is still no urine output. Lasix conversion PO→IV is 2: 1 while Bumex (bumetanide) is 1: 1 because it has good bioavailability & GI absorption.

4. **Assess the potential need for intubation** regardless of the SOB etiology (incase of severe hypoxia/ tachycardia). A BiPAP trial may be a helpful method of temporizing while talking to an upper level or waiting for MICU consultation.

   - BiPAP is most helpful to correct ventilation deficits (i.e. helps reduce pCO_2), especially in pts w/ CHF or COPD, but can assist any pt to help move air
   - BiPAP can be started at 15/5 & can be titrated as needed. Top number refers to IPAP (Inspiratory Positive Airway Pressure) while bottom number refers to EPAP (Expiratory PAP, equivalent to PEEP). You will also need to set the respiratory rate & FiO_2.
   - BiPAP is contraindicated in pts who are at risk of aspiration, on tube feeds, have excessive secretions, AMS, or respiratory arrest

(remember the contraindications to BiPAP, as you will see this quite often during your training).

5. Once you have the pt stabilized & have the results of your initial studies, you can initiate therapy directed at the specific etiology of the pt's dyspnea.

6. Congestive heart failure (CHF)

CHF pts usually present w/ SOB, particularly on exertion, mostly from volume overload & ↑ intra-ventricular filling pressures & can present with:

- **SOB or DOE**
- Generalized or lower extremity **edema**/ascites & weight gain,
- **Rales** on lung examination due to pulm congestion/edema,
- **Orthopnea** (ask how many pillows pt uses), & **paroxysmal nocturnal dyspnea** (PND).
- **Jugular venous distention** (JVD)
- **S3 gallop** on heart auscultation,

Two CHF types

1. **Systolic:** which is predicted by reduced EF (normal >55%)
2. **Preserved EF (or diastolic):** when the EF is normal but the pt has Sx of CHF w/ impaired relaxation. TTE is essential for diagnosis.

Etiology

For ↓ EF CHF: etiology is either ischemic (from CAD) or non-ischemic (broad spectrum DDx but most common cause is HTN). Left heart cath (or stress testing in low risk pts) to assess any reversible CAD is usually the first step in evaluating the cause for newly diagnosed heart failure (out pt process usually/cardiology call).

After ruling out obstructing CAD, then non-ischemic causes can be considered like HTN, structural heart problem (valvular disease), diabetes, obesity, toxins like alcohol (mostly large amount around 5-6 beers a day for more than 5 years), arrhythmias (tachycardia induced cardiomyopathy), volume overload from renal failure (insufficient dialysis), anemia, systemic infx, thyroid problems, COPD or pulm embolism (↑ right side afterload), amyloidosis, hemochromatosis, etc.

Preserved EF heart failure
The most common reason is prolonged uncontrolled HTN, & that is why it is sometimes called hypertensive heart disease (LVH on TTE or EKG can give a clue about uncontrolled HTN). Impair relaxation & pseudonormalization (more severe) are echo terms prescribing diastolic failure.

Management
- **CXR:** to check for pulm vascular congestion/edema, effusions, & cardiomegaly (chronic CHF pts may NOT have pulm edema but they still have CHF exacerbation; weight gain & JVD are clues)
- **EKG:** to check for sinus tachycardia, LVH, atrial & ventricular arrhythmia
- **Oximeter +/- ABG:** to check for hypoxia & respiratory alkalosis
- **TTE:** to distinguish systolic from diastolic dysfunction (may NOT need to have new TTE if pt already had one recently & Sx still the same)
- **Labs:** BNP to distinguish from non-cardiac SOB (BNP<100→ low suspicion, BNP>500→↑ suspicion). CMP to check for end organ damage due to hypoperfusion (liver & kidney).

Attention: checking BP is very important at the time of cardiac pulmonary edema presentation, as it will direct the duration/amount of diuresis.

Very high BP w/o peripheral edema may NOT need more than 2-3 liters net negative diuresis (HTN urgency → control BP is the issue) while **normal/low BP** w/ severe peripheral edema (due to maybe diuresis non-adherence) will need much more diuresis (fluid overload is the issue)

Acute treatment

Acute pulm edema is a common manifestation for decompensated CHF (diagnosed clinically w/ rales on auscultation/respiratory distress/desating/CXR later) & is treated by **LMNOP:** Lasix IV, Morphine PRN (w/caution due to sedating effect), Nitrates, O_2, & Position (sitting up on the bed to ↓ preload) along w/ maximizing CHF meds.

> **Attention:** controlling heart rate and BP is essential for pts w/ diastolic dysfunction as well as keeping them Euvolemic w/diuresis.

Chronic treatment of systolic dysfunction (EF <50%) is based on the use of **ACE inhibitors, β blockers, hydralazine w/ isosorbide dinitrate & spironolactone.** **Diuretics** are also used but have NOT been proven to lower mortality. **Digoxin** is used to ↓Sx & ↓ frequency of hospitalizations but has NOT been shown to ↓ mortality. **ACE inhibitors** can be used interchangeably w/ **ARBs.** The two common **β blockers** w/ evidence for lowering mortality in CHF are metoprolol & carvedilol (Bisoprolol does but NOT commonly used). ACE inhibitors & β blockers are indicated for CHF pts w/ systolic dysfunction at any stage of disease. **Spironolactone** lowers mortality for more advanced, Symptomatic disease, NYHA III-IV (should be added after maximizing β blocker & ACEi/ARB doses). Eplerenone is also K sparing diuretic, which is specifically good for CHF post MI (↓ mortality). Any pt originally presenting w/ pulm edema should get spironolactone.

Consider **intracardiac defibrillator (ICD)** when EF is <35% (for non-ischemic & <30% for ischemic cardiomyopathy) for more than 3 months on optimal medical Tx to prevent possible serious arrhythmias (mortality benefit due to primary prevention). ICD for primary prevention is usually an out pt process (when life expectancy is >1 year). If EF improved from reperfusion (from stents or CABG) or optimal medical therapy → no need for ICD.

Chronic treatment of diastolic dysfunction (preserved EF) is reliably treated w/ diuretics. However, you have to be careful NOT to overuse them. Benefit of β blocker & ACE inhibitors for diastolic dysfunction is NOT clear but they can be used to control BP (on rest & exertion) & heart rate (especially in case of A fib). Digoxin & spironolactone definitely do NOT help diastolic dysfunction (as for now but investigations are ongoing)

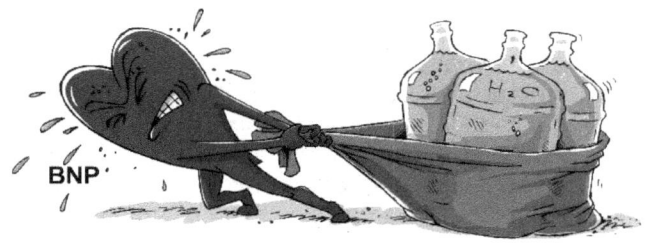

Heart failure (systolic/diastolic) is most often a struggle w/ fluid overload. Assess fluid status & diurese as needed.

Special consideration

- Left & right CHF is another heart failure classification. The left CHF is the common one & it can cause consequently right HF. Right HF can be the primary problem & manifest as LE edema, hepatocongestion, hepatojugular reflex, & ascites. Common etiology is pulm HTN, which can be assessed better by TTE or even right cardiac cath (to assess pulm artery resistance & effectiveness of Tx w/ med like sildenafil).

- Common **CHF exacerbation triggers** is non-compliance w/: meds (especially diuresis), low Na diet, fluid restriction, adjusting diuretic doses to the daily weight, dialysis (ESRD pts on dialysis). Another triggers: acute illness/infection, ischemia & iatrogenic (meds changes).
- "**Quick assessment**" for CHF: assess volume status, "wet or dry" to direct your diuretics management (like pulm edema, peripheral edema & JVD) & assess perfusion status "cold or warm" to direct your admission to the floor or ICU (extremities temperature, peripheral capillary perfusion). For "cold & dry or cold & wet", admit to the ICU for possible inotropic drip (like milrinone).
- For in pt management of **acute CHF exacerbation**, we generally start diuretic therapy w/ IV furosemide for 24-48h & then switch to PO form (& discharge when pt is Euvolemic). Consider switching to torsemide or bumetanide if the response to furosemide is inadequate. We can also try to use metolazone w/ loop diuretics (usually 30 minutes before the loop diuretics) to treat refractory edema because of the synergistic effect (monitor Mg & K closely). Always have a target for diuresis & urine output to achieve net fluid balance of negative ~1L/day & titrate the diuretic dose up & down accordingly. Consider HD/ultrafiltration to take fluid off for ESRD pts w/ CHF (as most of the time they do NOT make urine).
- Note that in pts w/ chronic kidney disease, ↓ glomerular filtration rate (GFR) is associated w/ ↑ plasma BNP. Also note that obese pts tend to have "pseudo" lower plasma BNP than non-obese pts (BNP dissolve in fat). Do NOT follow up BNP results to direct diuresis (did NOT show to help). Get BNP just on admission & before

discharge (BNP when pt is almost dry/Euvolemic for comparison in the future).

- If a pt presents w/ CHF exacerbation & is already on β blocker, you should ↓ dose by 50% temporarily in the acute phase; & if NOT on β blocker, you do NOT start it until the acute exacerbation resolves.
- Metoprolol succinate & Carvedilol (cheaper) are equal efficacy for LV dysfunction (↓ EF). Sometimes BP is at the low normal (like 100s, systolic) & Pt can NOT tolerate Coreg (due to alpha antagonist effect). In this scenario metoprolol will be a good alternative.
- **All CHF pts need close follow up** by cardiology or PCP W/ in 1 week to evaluate volume status & reconcile meds (as hospitals will NOT be reimbursed for readmission w/in 30 days from discharge). They also need to weigh themselves & call their doctor if there is weight gain more than 2-3lbs in 2days or 5lbs in 1 week (or pt simply can ↑ their diuresis dose as instructed like taking an extra tab) as intervention when these conditions are met has shown improved survival.
- **Pts w/ end-stage refractory CHF** (on optimal meds w/ NYHA class III- IV & >2-3 CHF admissions in 6 months) are candidates for extraordinary forms of therapy (LVAD or heart transplant) or for compassionate end-of-life care due to poor prognosis. High-risk feature for CHF: tachycardia, HoTN, worsening kidney function, ↑ liver enzymes/coagulopathy, ↑ lactic acid & AMS.

- **New York Heart Association NYHA** to assess exercise intolerance to know the severity of the CHF & direct the Tx.

Class 1	No physical limitation from CHF
Class II	Sx w/ ordinary activity (mild)
Class III	Sx w/ less than ordinary (minimal) activity like walking short distance or changing clothes but NOT on rest (moderate)
Class IV	Sx on rest (severe)

CHF Sx: fatigue, palpitation, dyspnea, or anginal pain.
Ordinary activity: is what a healthy person able to do like running, walking, climbing stairs, etc w/o CHF Sx.

7. Coronary Artery Disease (CAD)

The #1 cause of death in the USA & the world.

Cause
Atherosclerotic plaques in coronary arteries w/ some degree of obstruction. Usual intervention is w/ balloon/stents/CABG for lesions or stenosis>70% of the lumen of a large artery (LAD, RCA, diagonal, etc). Coronary ischemia is due to an imbalance between blood supply & O_2 demand, leading to inadequate perfusion.

Risk factors
Elevated LDL, ↓ HDL, smoking, HTN, DM, renal disease (especially Hemodialysis), genetics (family hx, especially 1st degree relative of male <55 or women <65), age (men over 45, women over 55), obesity, & sedentary life style.

Symptoms
Chronic or stable angina usually occurs w/ exercise or emotion (usually lasts <15 minutes & is relieved w/ rest or nitroglycerin). Typical Ischemic CP can be associated w/ SOB (most common), N/V, diaphoresis, & radiation of pain to left arm, neck or scapula. Unstable angina (consider ACS) occurs at rest (& also if the angina is new or ↑ chronic angina frequency/severity→ unstable angina). CAD (especially >60 years old) have no active Sx (which means that the lesions are NOT large enough to cause Sx usually >70% stenosis but they are still at risk of plaque ruptures & STEMI). For full work up of CP please see chapter under CP.

Diagnosis
- **Resting EKG:** look for Q waves (prior MI), any ST segment or T wave abnormalities, R wave progression & new AV blocks (new LBBB is

STEMI equivalent). Normal EKG during the chest pain is maybe reassuring but still does NOT r/o ACS (it is better to have more than one EKG; w/ & w/o CP). Make sure that the EKG changes are new comparing to a previous one as most of EKG ischemic changes can be normal variants if they are existed on previous ones

- **Exercise stress test** (if capable of walking on treadmill for 5-10 minutes): stress EKG or stress TTE. Stress test should NOT be done in the acute setting. Either at the same hospitalization (after r/u MI) or in few days after discharge as an out pt (in case of risk factors & moderate pretest probability for CAD)
- **Pharmacological stress test** for those who can NOT tolerate exercise stress test: IV adenosine, dipyridamole, or dobutamine can be used as cardiac stress inducing agents, which can be combined w/ an EKG, TTE, or Nuclear Perfusion Imaging.
- **Percutaneous Coronary Angiography PCA**: most sensitive test, used in pts being considered for revascularization (Percutaneous Transluminal Coronary Angioplasty (PTCA) or Coronary Artery Bypass Grafting (CABG)

Management
- Please refer to chest pain chapter for the **acute management.** Below is the chronic management, including secondary prevention.
- **Lifestyle modifications:** smoking cessation (can cut risk of CAD in half one year after smoking cessation), weight loss, diet & exercise (reduced intake of saturated fats & cholesterol)
- **Blood pressure control** in pts w/ HTN, goal: <130/90
- **Strict glycemic control** in pts w/ DM, goal A1C <6.5 (unless elderly w/ multiple comorbidities & risk for Hypoglycemia, goal A1C 7-8).

- **Medical therapy:** ASA, β blockers, Ca channels blockers, Statins, as well as Nitrates (either short acting like NTG tab/spray or long acting like Isosorbide mononitrate –Imdur-). In pts w/ recent stent placement, make sure they are taking additional ADP platelet receptor blocker such as Plavix (clopidogrel) or Effient (prasugrel) for at least 6 weeks (preferred up to 6 months-1year) for Bare-Metal Stent BMS & 1 year for Drug-Eluting Stent (DES).
- **Some lesions are NOT amenable to any intervention** (small artery, very distal, too many, etc) & medical therapy is the only option. End stage CAD is a term for CAD pts NOT candidate for intervention & failed medical therapy to control the CP.
- **Ranolazine (Ranexa):** is a "2nd line" anti-anginal meds for chronic angina & ↑ exercise tolerance by unknown mechanism, which is usually used after using the "1st line" anti-anginal meds (like β blockers, Ca channels blockers, & NTG) with persisting angina Sx. Do NOT use in hepatic impairment & adjust dose in renal impairment.
- **Revascularization** in pts w/ significant (>70%) coronary blockages:
  A. PCA: Coronary stents are now almost universally used in PCI procedures, often following balloon angioplasty, which opens the narrowed artery & facilitates stent placement
  B. CABG: for 3 or more vessels blockage (including left main or LAD) or any lesions are NOT amenable to stents. Some CAD lesions are NOT amenable for PCI or CABG (too many stenosis, no good graft target for CABG, small vessel disease, etc)

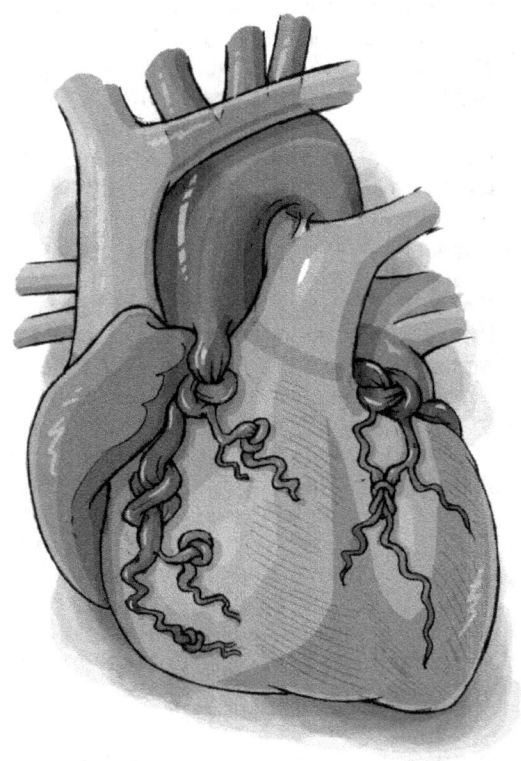

CAD is a common disease. Cardiac disease is the #1 cause of death worldwide.

Special considerations

- **Women & diabetics usually present w/ atypical symptoms** like N/V, abdominal pain, SOB or just generalized fatigue. Do NOT think about ACS only w/ CP.
- **Rule out MI** is a general term for pts who present w/ typical or atypical CP but they have negative troponin x1 & EKG is NOT ischemic. Admission may be warranted for observation to r/o ACS by serial troponin (usually q6hrs) & EKG

(if CP reoccur). Starting heparin drip or weight base dose lovenox is may be indicated for pts w/ high suspicion of ACS (like hx of MIs, typical CP, multiple risk factors, etc). Sometimes pts w/ low suspicion of ACS are admitted for serial troponins & EKG w/o starting heparin (depends on clinical judjement)

> **Attention:** Some pts has significant incompliant history w/ meds or diet or physician visits; placing Drug Eluting Stents DES is may be very dangerous due to the in-stent stenosis & thrombosis risk if they did NOT take palvix (medical management is better than stents; no need for heart cath).

- **Demand ischemia (or type 2 NSTEMI)** manifest by troponin elevation w/o plaque rupture (& intracoronary thrombosis like in ACS which is usually treated by heparin/balloon/stents). ↑ Cardiac O2 demand which results by ischemia occur in: sepsis, any infx, bacteremia, tachycardia for any reason, severe HTN or HoTN, Hypoxia or anemia (& basically anything will cause "cardiac stress"). **No indication (most of the time) for urgent PCA, especially w/ an active infx.** Although demand ischemia is well known but it is somewhat hard to diagnose & based on speculation; some pts will still have heart cath & it will be non-obstructive (usually troponin elevation is NOT very high, <1). **Prognosis:** is still poor w/ any troponin elevation even w/o coronary obstruction/thrombosis (↑ mortality similar to the "real" NSTEMI, type 1).
- **Cocaine:** do NOT start & even stop β blockers in case of cocaine use (contraindicated due to refractory HTN). The use of β blockers may exacerbate the vasospasm induced by cocaine

due to an "unopposed alpha 1 effect" which may cause a significantly elevated systemic blood pressure.

- Around 40% of sudden death from ACS occurred from **plaque rupture** in pts with even 30-50% stenosis "non-obstructive lesions" which do NOT indicate PCI (balloon/stents). Therefore, 90% lesions (which may cause angina symptoms) may NOT cause mortality as the 30% lesions as the later has higher % to rupture due to the high blood flow status, which can cause fibrous cap erosion and, subsequent, rupture. This makes the whole preop evaluation & risk stratification maybe questionable.

- **Anginal equivalent:** acute induction or worsening of diastolic dysfunction by ischemia raises left atrial & pulm venous pressure. This explains why many patients with coronary heart disease have respiratory symptoms with their anginal pain, including wheezing, an inability to take a deep breath, SOB, & even overt pulm edema. These respiratory symptoms can occur in the absence of anginal pain & are often referred to as **"anginal equivalents."**

- **TIMI score:** is a very useful tool to assess the risk for ACS (& ask targeted Qs for complete H & P) & help in the decision of "is the CP ischemic or not?" Including TIMI score in your assessment help to quickly estimate the ACS risk.

Age 65 years old or older	1 point
Aspirin used in the last 7 days	1 point
Angina occurred 2 or more times in the last 24 hours	1 point
ST changes 0. 5mm or more on admit EKG	1 point
Serum Troponin or other biomarker elevated	1 point
Coronary Artery Disease history (w/ at least 50% Coronary Artery stenosis)	1 point
Cardiac Risk Factors w/ at least 3 present (e.g. Hypertension, Hyperlipidemia, premature CAD Family History, Tobacco abuse)	1 point

Total score 0-1: 4.7% risk
Total score 2: 8.3% risk
Total score 3: 13.2% risk
Total score 4: 19.9% risk
Total score 5: 26.2% risk
Total score 6-7: 40.9% risk

8. Hypertension (HTN)

Primary HTN

Normal blood pressure		Systolic <120 mmHg & diastolic <80 mmHg
PreHTN		Systolic 120 to 139 mmHg or diastolic 80 to 89 mmHg
HTN	Stage 1	Systolic 140 to 159 mmHg or diastolic 90 to 99 mmHg.
	Stage 2	Systolic ≥160 or diastolic ≥100 mmHg

Management
Lifestyle modifications & drug therapy. Consider Na restriction, weight loss, dietary modification, exercise, & relaxation techniques. If lifestyle modifications have no effect over 3-6 months→initiate medical therapy (initiate meds if stage 2 directly)

Tx:
Consider comorbidities & drug adverse effects (DAE):
- **Thiazide diuretics** such as HCTZ or chlorthalidone (better than HCTZ) are very common. DAE: hyponatremia, ↑ Ca reabsorption (prevent osteoporosis) & ↑ uric acid reabsorption (worsen gout) in the kidney.
- **Diabetes:** use ACE-I/ARB (like lisinopril/losartan) as it protects the kidney & helps w/ proteinuria. DAE: AKI (in pts w/ CKD), ↑ K, cough, angioedema (tongue/throat/face swelling w/ SOB). Do NOT use if Cr>2. 5-3 or in renal artery stenosis. Monitor BMP (Cr & K) more frequent

when you first start ACEi/ARB (↑ in Cr <30% of baseline is expected due to the mechanism of action & meds should NOT be stopped just because of that). ACEi/ARB are contraindicated in pregnancy (do NOT prescribe if pt is trying to conceive, category D)

- **CAD:** use β blocker (metoprolol either short acting like titrate q12h or succinate q24h, atenolol, Coreg)
- **CHF:** use β blocker, ACE-I or ARB (if ACE-I is NOT tolerated, use ARB)
- **Migraine:** β blocker or CCB (it has prophylactic effects)
- **Hyperthyroidism:** β blocker (Propranolol)
- **Osteoporosis:** thiazide (because it reabsorbsCa) & avoid thiazide in gout (reabsorbs uric acid)
- **Pregnancy:** alpha methyldopa, labetalol, CCB, Clonidine (rebound HTN is common in case of sudden stoppage), thiazide diuretics & hydralazine (used IV for preeclampsia)
- **BPH:** alpha blocker (Prazosin or flomax)

If BP is NOT controlled w/ one drug, add a second drug: β blocker, ACE-I/ARB, CCB, sprinolactone, thiazide
If BP is still NOT controlled w/ the second drug, add a third drug (include diuretics if NOT already) & investigate for secondary HTN causes (preferably after 24 hrs continues BP monitor to confirm elevated BP).

Secondary HTN
Investigate for secondary HTN if you see the following: Young (<30) or old (>60) pt, refractory HTN (failure to control w/ 3 meds including diuretics), Bruit (renal artery stenosis), Episodic HTN (pheochromocytoma), Buffalo hump, truncal obesity, striae (Cushing's), Hypokalemia (Conn's), UE pressure>LE pressure (coarctation of the aorta), & Hirsutism (congenital adrenal hyperplasia)

Special considerations:

- **Start w/ two anti HTN meds** for pts w/ Stage 2 HTN & adjust doses in following visits (usually one med is NOT enough).
- **Check BP multiple times** (do NOT diagnose HTN from single reading), no caffeine, empty bladder, no tobacco or EtOH, relaxed, sitting down & try different devices if error suspected (or manually).
- **Every effort should be done to put pts on β blocker & ACE-I/ARB** due to the great mortality benefits they offer to diabetic & CHF pts. Escalate the doses as tolerated & check the heart rate for the β blocker (do NOT escalate if HR around 60) & the serum Cr for ACE-I.
- **Elderly Pts** especially w/ long-term DM & ESRD (stiff arteries due to calcification) experience hypotensive Sx on normal systolic BP readings like 110s-120s. De-escalate BP meds to achieve "new normal BP" in the range of 140s-150s.
- **HTN Emergency:** BP >210s/120s w/ end organ damage (like AMS, AKI, elevated liver enzymes, pulm edema) needs immediate action w/ IV drip meds like NTG, Na nitroprusside, Labetalol/ Esmolol, Nicardipine & fenoldopam. PO meds can also be used like Hydralazin &/or Clonidine while waiting for the drip.
- **HTN urgency** (same as emergency but no end organ damage) can be managed on the floor w/ PO agents like nitropaste (topical), hydralazine, Clonidine, captopril (short acting NOT lisinopril which is long acting) & labetalol. Do NOT ↓ BP more than 25% in the 1st 6 hrs (could cause cerebral hypoperfusion). Non-compliance w/ HTN meds (especially Clonidine & β blocker) is a common reason for extreme HTN.
- **Elevated BP can be caused by CNS problems** like CVA or elevated intra-cranial pressure (ICP). Do NOT ↓ systolic BP <140s-150s in the 1st 1-2 days

- **Chronic NSAID** use causes/worsens HTN. Switch to Tylenol if possible.

> **Attention**: decongestants OTC that contain ephedrine could cause worsening HTN → HTN urgency/emergency. Always review new meds for worsening HTN.

- **Thiazides** ↑ serum Ca (& uric acid), whereas **furosemide** ↓ Ca.
- **Controlling BP is very essential** for systolic & diastolic CHF Tx (afterload reduction)
- ↓ **PO intake** is a problem for pt w/ HTN as most of the meds are PO & IV HTN meds is NOT recommended in the floor (mostly in the ICU). Clonidine patches are a good option.

9. Atrial Fibrillation (a fib)

A fib is a tachycardia heart arrhythmia that is important to recognize on monitor & EKG & be able to effectively treat & manage. A fib is either new onset or recurrent. Paroxysmal A fib happens sporadically (self-limiting, intermittent) or persistent (>7days). The main three problems are: Loss of atrial contraction→CHF Sx; left atrium stasis→ thromboemboli; tachycardia→tachycardia induced cardiomyopathy (usually in hours-days)

Common Etiologies of A fib

Hyperthyroid, pulm embolism, Cardiac ischemia, CHF, Mitral valve disease, post surgeries (↑ catecholamine status), Anemia, EtOH (holiday heart), HTN, old age & stimulants (caffeine, amphetamine, cocaine). Try to treat the underlying etiology while treating a fib (if possible).

Clinical features
1. Palpitations, dizziness, angina, or syncope.
2. Fatigue & dyspnea on exertion.
3. Irregularly irregular pulse.
4. CVA (from thrombus embolus to brain)

Evaluation
1. Obtain 12 lead EKG & compare to prior EKG if necessary (old or new).
2. Hx of any previous heart arrhythmias (any palpitations, pre/syncope), hx of OSA, recent surgery or trauma (high catecholamine status).
3. Physical exam: cardiac auscultation (irregular irregularity), check peripheral pulses, JVD, presyncope, DOE.
4. TTE (check L atrium enlaregment, valvular disease, or clots?), & thyroid function.

Management
- **Check vitals (ACLS for unstable pts).** Unstable pts should undergo immediate synchronized

electrical cardioversion (do NOT wait for TTE or anticoagx). Instability is defined as SBP<90, acute Congestive heart failure, pulm edema, confusion, or CP.

- **Stable pts should have their heart rate slowed** if it is >100-110. You can achieve that w/ rate control meds, which are β Blockers PO or IV up to q6h (metoprolol), Ca channel blockers Po or IV (diltiazem), or digoxin (last resort due to toxicity & low efficiency comparing to the other agents). Consider cardioversion w/ either rhythm control medicine (Amiodarone is commonly used to medically convert the rhythm to sinus & also can control the rate) or electrocardioversion (especially if you want to keep the atrial kick in case of CHF, pulm edema, or HoTN); usually it is a cardiology call. All drips are usually used in ICU setting. **Digoxin:** NOT commonly used anymore but can control the rate only at rest (↑ parasympathic activity but NOT effect sympathic pathway).

> **Attention:** No clear survival benefits from rhytm control (sinus) vs rate control. In general: cardioversion is maybe preferred for 1st onset (better <7days, the earlier the better), unstable, active CHF (to keep the "atrial kick").
> **Attention:** Anticoagulate all pts (regardless of CHADS2 core) after cardioversion for 4-12 weeks as the atria is mechanically stunned and also high risk for recurrence in 1st three months.

- **Acute decompenstated CHF & a fib w/ RVR is a hard combination** to treat as AV blocking agents like β blocker & CCB are needed to control the HR but they will worsening the CHF; call cardiology. **Few options to consider:** DC cardioversion, amiodarone IV bolus/drip/PO (control heart rate as well as ability to convert the rhythm to sinus), & digoxin (IV or PO).

- **Consider Transesophageal Echocardiography (TEE)** to r/o left atrium thrombosis if you want to cardiovert a fib if it occurred >48hours (hard to assess if pt is NOT on telemetry monitoring) & pt is stable (cardiovert unstable pts regardless).

> **Attention:** No need for TEE for pts fully anticoagulated (INR 2-3) for >3-4 weeks. If pt had atrium clots→ delay cardioversion until the clots resolve with anticoagx (to prevent CVA).

- **Check & replace Mg & K** trying to keep Mg above 2 & K above 4.
- **Consider PO anticoagx** depending on CHADS2 score to prevent stroke (risk is usually 3-4% per year & depends on CHADS2 score). Make sure that there is no contraindication like active bleeding or previous recent hemorrhagic strokes when you start anticoagx.
- **AV node ablation & pacemaker:** is a last resort for a fib w/ RVR.
- **CHADS2** is a scoring system to indicate the need for anticoagx & can be calculated as CHF 1 pnt, HTN 1 pnt, Age>75 1 pnt, Diabetes 1 pnt, or Stroke/TIA 2 pnts. PO anticoagx are either warfarin or any of the newer agents like Dabigatran (Pradaxa), Apixaban Eliquis) or rivaroxaban (Xarelto) which are expensive (ensurance companies may NOT cover them). **CHADS2:**
Score 0 → ASA (325mg). Check CHA2D2-VASc to make sure that the score is really low.
Score 1→ either just ASA or ASA + PO anticoagx. Also check VASc

Score ≥2 → PO anticoagx (no need for ASA unless indicated for another reason). No need for VASc as anticoagx is obviously indicated.

- **CHA2D2-VASc:** is another scoring system which maybe better for females (**available online**).
- **HAS-BLED:** is another scoring system to calculate major bleeding risk which can also guide the decision of starting anticaogx for a fib pts (**available online**)

10. Asthma & COPD

Common cause of SOB & DOE associated w/ allergy for asthma & smoking for COPD. Usually wheezing is very suggestive of asthma/COPD.

PFTs findings in pt w/ Asthma & COPD:

FEV1 is ↓ & FVC is usually normal → ↓ FEV1/FVC *ratio (reversible in Asthma after bronchodilator but NOT in COPD).*

*↑ **in residual volume** (more in COPD).*

*↓ **in DLCO** caused by destruction of lung interstitium, which is mainly in COPD; especially emphysema (can be normal or high in asthma).*

Exam
Chest (wheezing, PNA signs, pulm edema), heart (CHF signs, gallops, murmurs), extremity (cyanosis, edema, warm), & neurological (AMS from hypoxia).

Management
O_2 & ABG, CXR, Albuterol (inhaled/jet neb) +/- ipratropium, bolus of steroids (usually PO prednisone 40-80mg daily). If fever, sputum, & /or new infiltrate are present on CXR, add ceftriaxone & azithromycin for community-acquired PNA.

Chronic management for asthma
- Start w/ short acting bronchodilator **(albuterol) prn** as rescue meds (for mild Asthma; 1st line Tx).
- If NOT controlled, add a chronic controller meds such as an **inhaled steroid (low dose** or you can step up to **moderate dose** for better control). You can start w/ controller +rescue meds prn if asthma is moderate or severe
- If inhaled albuterol prn & inhaled steroids moderate dose did NOT control Sx (pt is still using albuterol often at the day & wake up at night w/ SOB) add **long acting inhaled beta agonist LABA such as salmeterol or formoterol**. Using

long acting beta agonist w/o inhaled steroid in asthma pts ↑ mortality (but NOT for COPD).
- **PO steroids** are a last resort

Steps in chronic management of COPD
1. Tiotropium or ipratropium inhaler w/ or w/o Albuterol inhaler (as monotherapy)
2. Add long acting inhaled beta agonist LABA such as salmeterol or formoterol.
3. Add inhaled steroids.
4. Add PO steroids (also consider cardiopulm rehabilitation).

For last stages, consider surgical options such as LVRS & lung transplantation.

Attention: LABA can be added before inhaled steroids in asthma pts (but NOT in COPD)

Pneumococcal vaccine & annual influenza vaccine, smoking cessation (improves mortality).
Long-term home O_2 if the **PO_2 < 56** or **O_2 sat <88 %** (improves mortality).

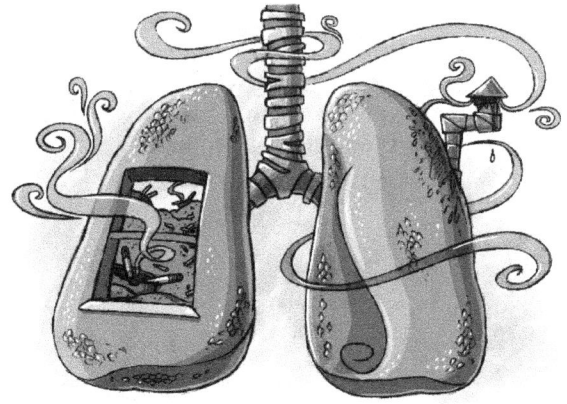

Smoking is #1 preventable cause for COPD.

Special considerations

- Asthma or COPD exacerbation pts who can NOT talk full sentence from their SOB need immediate action by administer O_2 & jet neb (albuterol & ipratropium), IV steroid (methylprednisolone) & possible urgent ICU evaluation (for possible intubation) while awaiting ABG & CXR results. ↑ CO_2 is a sign of imminent respiratory failure from possible respiratory muscle weakness & decompensation.

> **Attention:** β blocker is NOT contraindicated for pts w/ mild to moderate controlled COPD & benefits may out-weigh risks for cardiac indications to use.

- **Consider adjunctive therapy:** like Montelukast or theophylline as indicated
- **Assess severity of the COPD/asthma** w/ FEV1 results: >80% is mild, 80-50% is moderate, 49-30% is severe, <30% is very severe (consider palliative/hospice care evaluation if Symptomatic, on home O_2 & refractory to all meds).
- **Inhaled meds are essential in COPD management;** if a pt is NOT responding to therapy, therapy adherence should be verified & inhaler technique (**available online**) should be assessed before therapy is adjusted (consider spacer to improve inhalation especially for children & dementia pts).

11. Pneumonia (PNA)

PNA is a very common cause for hospital admissions. Knowing how to appropriately recognize & treat PNA is an essential part of internal medicine.

Signs & symptoms
Fever, cough, sputum (yellowish/greenish in bacterial & even viral infx), pleuritic CP, dyspnea, & tachypnea

Work-up
Hx, vitals, physical exam (crackles on auscultation, egophony, tactile fremitus), CXR (infiltration & opacities sometimes are hard to notice & differentiate them from atelectasia), sputum/blood cultures, Strep urine antigen, CBC w/ differential, BMP, & other labs as pertinent (legionella antigen, fungal cultures, respiratory panel, LDH); pleural thoracentesis & bronchoscopy (BAL) if indicated.

Pneumonia Types & Management

- **Community Acquired Pneumonia (CAP):** Pneumonia acquired outside of medical facility that does NOT fit in the definition of HCAP. Standard out pt therapy is monotherapy w/ a fluoroquinolone (Levaquin) or Augmentin + Azithromycin. In hospital setting, start Ceftriaxone/Azithromycin IV.
- **Healthcare Associated Pneumonia (HCAP):** Criteria include hospitalization in acute care hospital for two or more days in last 90 days, residence in nursing home or long-term care facility in last 30 days, receiving out pt IV therapy or home wound care in last 30 days, or attending hospital clinic or dialysis center w/ in 30 days. Also included PNA that begins 48-72 hrs after hospital admission. Standard abx are Vanc & Zosyn IV (covers G+, G-, & anaerobic including MRSA &

Pseudomonas) as initial therapy. Tailor therapy according to C & S.

- **Ventilator Associated Pneumonia (VAP):** PNA occurring after 48 hrs of pt being intubated & placed on mechanical ventilation. Tx is same as for HCAP (must cover Pseudomonas).

Special considerations

- **Community Acquired PNA Risk Stratification:** good standard guide for admission is **CURB-65:** Confusion, Uremia (BUN >20), Respiratory rate >30, Blood pressure <90/60, Age >65. Score of 0-1: out pt. Score of 2: in pt. Score of 3 or greater: assess for ICU.
- **There are many types of PNA**: bacterial, viral (self-limited/supportive management/Tamiflu in 48hrs), fungal (certain places & immunocompromised pts) causes but this is a good guide for initial management.
- **PNA can be hard to diagnose clinically** for some pts especially CHF pts (BNP may help) & more testing is needed (CXR or chest CT scan). Atelectasis on CXR can look similar to infiltration, which is the cornerstone objective sign for PNA diagnosis. Correlate w/ the clinical picture & do NOT feel obligated to a full course of abx if PNA was misdiagnosed.

> **Attention:** Repeat CXR in 12-24hrs (for comparison) as PNA infiltration unlikely to resolve but atelectasis or fluid edema may do (especially if diuresis is given).

12. Hemoptysis

Expectoration of blood from lower respiratory tract; does NOT have to be accompanied by sputum production. Can range from blood-streaked sputum to massive expectoration & life-threatening bleeding. The amount of blood could be small but it is significant in the lungs (at that case, usually vitals are unstable w/ tachypnea, O_2 desaturation, & SOB).
If the source of expectorated blood is from upper respiratory tract/GI tract → pseudo hemoptysis. *Massive hemoptysis: acute, life-threatening bleeding defined as ≥500 mL/24hr or bleeding rate ≥100 mL/hr.*

Etiology
3B's → most common are bronchitis/PNA, bronchogenic CA, & bronchiectasis. Less common reasons: foreign body, airway trauma, Aspergilloma, CHF, Mitral Stenosis (MS), Pulm AVM, pulm embolism, TB, Wegener's Granulomatosis, good-pasture disease, coagulopathy: thrombocytopenia or anticoagx meds, complication of bronchoscopy or lung bx, & Cocaine (more of nasal bleeding from sniffing).

H & P
- Make sure it is a true hemoptysis, NOT just nasal or hematemesis
- Assess quantity, frequency, onset (acute or chronic), & presence of sputum
- Associated w/ SOB, fever, chills, & /or night sweats (infectious?)
- Diastolic heart murmur (for MS)
- Epistaxis, telangiectasias, renal insufficiency (for AVM & autoimmune etiology)
- Weight loss, cachexia, & smoker (malignancy)
- ASA, NSAIDS, & anticoagx

Tests:
- Pulse Ox, ABG, CXR
- CBC w/ diff, renal panel, UA
- Coagx status: PT/INR/PTT
- Sputum w/ gram stain & culture; acid fast stain, cytology
- ANA, ANCA, anti-GBM antibody
- BNP, TTE, high resolution CT
- Assess need for bronchoscopy w/ biopsy

Management

Massive hemoptysis
- Establish airway; if in respiratory distress, INTUBATE
- Transfuse blood products as needed: FFP, platelets, & pure RBC
- Bronchoscopy: balloon tamponade, iced saline lavage, topical vasoconstrictives (i.e. Epinephrine or topical thrombin), cautery, cryotherapy
- Angiography, embolization, & surgery

Stable hemoptysis
- Bed rest, supportive care w/ IV fluids, supplemental O_2, & serial CBCs. Treat underlying etiology. If you know the location of bleeding, make the pt turn toward the good lung to improve blood circulation & oxygenation.

13. GI bleed

Symptoms
- **Upper:** N/V, hematemesis, coffee ground emesis, epigastric pain, & melena (black tarry stool from digested blood).
- **Lower:** Diarrhea, tenesmus, bright red blood per rectum, hematochezia (note: bloody stool can also be seen in rapid upper GI bleeding, but usually vitals will NOT be stable).

Etiology/Tx

Upper GI bleed	1. Peptic ulcer	50%: NSAIDs intake is common, H. *pylori* & ↑ gastric PH. Tx: EGD for possible clip or cauterization as indicated along w/ IV PPI, such as esomeprazole for 72 hrs then switch to high dose PO PPI like omeprazole 40mg BID.
	2. Varices	10-30%: esophageal (or gastric) from portal HTN. Tx: EGD w/ banding, octreotide IV for 2-5 days & prophylactic abx if the pt has cirrhosis (either ceftriaxone IV or norfloxacin PO). Consider TIPS for refractory cases.

Upper GI bleed cont-	3. **Esophagitis, gastritis, & duodenitis**	25%: due to NSAIDs, ASA, GERD & other meds, such as bisphosphonates & doxycycline. Tx: d/c the offending agent (NSAID, ASA, etc) & start PPI or H2 antagonist.
	4. **Mallory-Weiss tear**	Located at the gastro-esophageal junction from retching & vomiting. Tx: usually self-limited, but consider EGD if bleeding continues.
Lower GI bleed	1.**Diverticulosis**	Very common. Tx: usually self-limited, but if NOT then consider colonoscopy (for epinephrine injection, banding, APC, cauterizing). Last resort is to consult IR for embolization or general surgery for resection of the bleeding segment.
	2. **Malignancy**	Usually it is occult blood (positive FOBT & iron deficiency anemia). Management: colonoscopy
	3. **Colitis**	IBD (UC>CD), infx, mesenteric ischemia. Tx: steroids, abx or surgery evaluation as indicated.

Lower GI bleed cont-	4.Angiodysplasia (AVM), hemorrhoids, & anal fissures:	Rectal exam is diagnostic sometimes. Tx: usually self-limited, otherwise consider colonoscopy for intervention (or consult IR for embolization or surgery for resection).

Management for both upper & lower bleeding

First step:
Assess blood loss by vitals (tachycardia at >10% volume loss, orthostatic HoTN at >20% loss, & shock at >30% loss).
Resuscitate by two large IV lines & bolus fluid (mostly normal saline) until vitals stabilize. Type & screen 2-8 units PRBC on hold to transfuse if Hgb<7, but that threshold may be higher if there are comorbidities like CAD. Check PT/PTT/INR & reverse them w/ FFP, vitamin K, or platelets (keep >50k).
Check for organ failure: including AMS, urine output, liver dysfunction, & SOB.
Consider ICU if the vitals do NOT normalize after 1-2 L of IV fluids or if the pt had organ failure (abnormal LFTs, high Cr, AMS, CHF, SOB, or ongoing bleeding).
For ongoing bleeding call GI for possible scope & intervention to stop the bleed. Consider general surgery evaluation for the unstable pt w/ ongoing bleeding for possible laparotomy & resection.

Second step
Ask about the use of the following: NSAIDs, ASA, anticoagulants, antiplatelet agents, alcohol abuse, previous GI bleed, liver disease, or coagulopathy.
Sx & signs: abdominal pain, hematemesis or "coffee ground" emesis, passing melena/tarry stool.
Examination: vital signs, rectal examination for stool

color (melena vs. hematochezia vs. brown), anal fissures or hemorrhoids, & guaiac testing.

> **Attention:** Significant abdominal tenderness accompanied by signs of peritoneal irritation (e.g. involuntary guarding) suggests perforation.

NG tube w/ lavage is informative & easy test to localize the bleeding (upper or lower) if the diagnosis is unknown or can also clean the stomach before EGD. If it is an active upper GI bleed there will be fresh blood; if recent bleed & some digestion of blood has occurred → it will be coffee grounds; if it is non-bloody bile, the source may be lower or the bleeding was missed.
Keep the pt NPO (advance diet to clear liquid after diagnosis & Tx as indicated). Assess the comorbidities (to know when to transfuse & triage the pt to ICU vs. floor).

Special considerations
- **GI bleeding is NOT painful by itself;** therefore, abdominal pain (especially w/ guarding) may indicate perforation (order erect abdominal x-ray or KUB looking for free air & consider a stat general surgery evaluation). Consider mesenteric ischemia for pain out of proportion to signs, & worse w/ eating. The bleeding may indicate necrosis (surgery evaluation for resection may be needed to prevent sepsis).
- **Blood has a bowel stimulant effect** & causes diarrhea, so constipated pts are unlikely to have GI bleed.
- **Upper GI bleed is 80% of the GI bleeding** (that is why an EGD/NG tube is maybe indicated if the source of bleeding is unknown). A high percentage of GI bleeds are self-limited & will stop

spontaneously, however you still need to evaluate & treat due to a high percentage of recurrence.

- **An NG tube is part of the initial management** but be aware that it is contraindicated for variceal bleeding, therefore a detailed hx about cirrhosis, variceal bleeds, & endoscopic intervention like clipping is essential.
- **For acute bleeding** (NOT just GI bleeds), Hgb level may be falsely normal in the 1st few hrs due to plasma shifting. Vital signs are reflective of blood volume status more than the Hgb number, especially in the 1st few hrs.
- **Transfuse RBC**, regardless of Hgb level, if vitals are unstable after attempted fluid resuscitation.
- **Obscure bleeding** accounts for approximately 5% of the bleeds: no cause is found by upper & lower endoscopy. Many etiologies may be present. Management: repeat EGD & colonoscopy w/ push to the duodenum & ileum, capsule swallow (repeat to high sensitivity), Tc99 scan, tagged RBC scan, & angiography.
- **Stop & /or reverse any anticoagx.** It may be resumed after the bleeding stops & appropriate intervention is performed. Sometimes you need to weigh the pros & cons depending on the reason of anticoagx.
- **PPI drip** (which is NOT the same as PO/IV PPI) is indicated for upper GI bleed & it need to be continued for 72 hrs after EGD only if ulcer is seen w/ active bleeding/oozing or an obvious vessel in the base of the ulcer (high % of rebleeding in this case).

14. Antibiotics (abx)

The best abx choice is to send a good culture specimen for sensitivity & choose the PO form (or the IV form at first & then switch to PO as indicated) w/ consideration of the side effect, expense, frequency, & comorbidity. You can follow up the infx resolution & the abx effectiveness by monitoring the fever, Sx, ESR/CPR, WBC & clinical improvement. <u>Know what you are treating</u>.

Common used abx

- **Vancomycin**: 1st line G + broad coverage, good for MRSA. IV form for broad coverage especially for sepsis or confirmed gram+ infx like strep & staph including MRSA. PO form is only for c diff infx as it does NOT absorb in GI track. Follow up blood troughs (usually after the 3rd dose) & adjust dose accordingly (therapeutic 15-20mcg/ml). Dosing is mostly BID for normal kidney but should be changed to either daily or q48hrs for AKI or CKD stage ≥ III (pharmacy can help dosing). On dialysis, give the dose after the session & get trough before it as 30% will be dialyzed out. Common empiric therapy w/ Zosyn.

- **Clindamycin:** gram + & anaerobic, PO for anaerobic infx mainly below the diaphragm like abscess, mild cellulitis out pt, aspiration PNA. Effective against community MRSA (althoughdoxycline & bactrim is better). Weak against group B strep & ↑risk of c. diff.

- **Daptomycin**: IV, Gram positive. Usually is NOT the 1st choice & is used when Vanc fails as it has great MRSA coverage. Do NOT use for respiratory infx (due to pulmonary surfactant inhibition effect on Daptomycin, but it is good for osteomyelitis & skin infx). Is NOT aminoglycoside.

- **Zosyn (Pipercellin/Tazobactam):** IV form, 1st line broad-spectrum coverage (Gram+, - & anerobic), for moderate & severe infx like nosocomial PNA, abdomen infx (diverticulitis, abscess & peritonitis), skin infx. Does NOT cover MRSA. Can be used w/ Amikacin (aminoglycoside) to cover nosocomial pseudomonas. Common combination w/ Vanc as empiric Tx.

Same group: Unasyn (Ampicillin/Sulbactam), which is good against G- in general (Unlike Zosyn; it does NOT cover Pseudomonase). Augmentin (Amoxicillin/Clavulanate) is PO & common for out-pt mild-moderate infx like bacterial pharyngitis & sinusitis, animal bites, mild cellulitis (including diabetic foot), lower respiratory infx, & pyelonephritis.

- **Rocephin (Ceftriaxone):** IV cephalosporin, 3rd G, broad coverage (G+ & -), weak against Pseudomonas & anaerobic (do NOT use). Does NOT cover enteroccus (All cephalosporins do NOT cover it) or MRSA. Used for meningitis (especially caused by S. Pneumonia or meningococcal), gonococcalinfx, & prophylactic after sexual assault, UTI, skin infx, pelvic inflammatory disease, bone infx, & CAP (in combination w/ azithromycin).

  Same Group: Ceftaroline: 5th G cephalosporin & covers all MRSA; even Vanc resistant. **Cefdinir & Cefixime:** PO 3rd G cephalosporins (good for out pt therapy)

- **Azithromycin (z pack):** common out pt PO abx for atypical PNA, bronchitis, & GPC. 5 tablets 250mg each in 4 days. 2tab 1st day & then once qdaily. Yellow greenish phlegm does NOT automatically mean z pack.

- **Keflex:** 1stG cephalosporin, PO for G +. Treats bone infx, UTI, otitis media, Upper RTI, strep pharyngitis. Mainly for skin flora & surgery likes them for prophylaxis. Great for cellulitis strep infx (good for MSSA).

  Same group: Ancef & Duricef

- **Linozolid:** PO or IV, Gram + including MRSA & Enterococcus. No Gram- coverage. Usually is a

2nd line after Vanc, especially for vanc resistance enterococcus. **Treat:** CAP, HCAP & skin infx. Does NOT treat bacteremia (NOT bactericidal).

- **Ciprofloxacin:** great for G- & pseudomonas (NOT good for G+). Used also for gastroparesis (from long lasting diabetes, manifests as early satiety & N/V) to ↑ GI motility. Prolongs QT interval. Use for: UTI, GI infx, CAP. Usually orally but available IV. Same group: Moxifloxacin & Levofloxacine (respiratory quinolones), which are preferred for CAP (good for G+ compared to Ciprofloxacin).
- **Amphotericin B:** IV, for severe fungal infx, mainly for AIDS & neutropenia pt or any immunosuppressed pt w/ presumed fungal infx for empiric fungal coverage. Order fungal blood culture before initiation. Nephrotoxic, hydration before & while on the med. Monitor electrolytes & kidney function.
- **Fluconazole:** common anti-fungal po drug for either Tx of common fungal infx especially candida (like PO thrush, vaginal candidiasis is, & even more severe cases like cryptococcal meningitis in AIDS) or prophylactic for immunosuppressed pts like in BMT. High doses can treat fungemia. Diflucan 150mg one dose po is a common Tx for vaginal candidiasis w/ white cheesy discharge (Vaginal Miconazole is another option). **Nystatin** is good for Candida infx like vaginal w/ creamy discharge, PO w/ white painful lesions or thrush, & skin candida (or Tania) w/ white flaky red skin w/ itching (use w/ combination of steroid like **Betamethasone** for Symptomatic relief). **Clotrimazole** topical is also effective against candida & most of other topical fungal infx (including athlete foot). Same group: **Voriconazol** (good for mold like aspergillus as fluconazole does NOT cover mold) & **Itraconazol**: for presumed serious fungal infx (comes in PO form).
- **Acyclovir:** effective against shingles if administered in 72 hrs from the blistering to

reduce pain & ↓ duration. Another indication: herpetic encephalitis & genital herpes. Hydrate well before & during Tx due to risk of AKI. Same group: **ganciclovir** (mainly for CMV infx)

- **Metronidazole (Flagyl):** anerobic, 1st choice for clostridium difficile infx, vaginal infx (vaginosis w/ thin fishy smelling discharge & trichomoniasis w/ greenish yellowish discharge), Colorecatal infx, Giardia & Amebia infx. Category B in pregnancy (A accepted, D life threatening). Avoid Alcohol & educate about metallic taste.

- **Amikacin:** Aminoglycoside IV covers G- mainly. Treat: UTI, meningitis (G- infx), HCAP including Pseudomonas respiratory infx. Have nephro, neuro, & ototoxicity side effects.
Same group: Gentamycin & Tobramycin (the best for pseudomonas & G-)

- **Doripenem:** broad coverage (GPC, GNB, & anerobic) except MRSA. From carbapenem group. Good for pseudomonas (intubation associated PNA or VAP). Only IV & is NOT usually 1st line Tx. Usually switched to it from zosyn if it fails for possible resistance (great gram negative coverage). At the same group: **Meropenem** which↑ risk of seizure in pt w/ CNS problem & **Ertapenem**, which is NOT covering pseudomonas but still good broad coverage (used once daily IV).

- **Aztreonam (monobactam abx):** IV/IM broad coverage for G- including pseudomonas aeruginosa (NOT good for G+ or anerobic). It is a synthetic monocyclic beta-lactam antibiotic (a monobactam). It is usually NOT the first line & used when other agents fail covering G- infx (like for UTI). Good option for penicillin allergy (cross reactivity is very low)

- **Bactrim:** Sulfa drug, usually PO. Very common use: PCP infx (& prophylactically) in immunosuppressed pts, UTI (lower for 3 days & upper use IV or PO for longer time, around 14days), skin (& soft tissue infx), CA-MRSA, &

COPD exacerbation. Caution w/ sulfa allergy & in pregnancy (category C).

Special considerations:

- **Good culture specimens**
  - ○ **Sputum:** Squamous epithelial cells line the mouth. If> 10 of these cells are present in the specimen then it is may be sputum w/ saliva but if<10 per hpf & >25 PMNs in the specimen, it is more likely to be from the lungs. Consider bronchoscopy by pulm for good sputum samples, if needed.
  - ○ **Urine:** mid-stream clean catch (foley cath is NOT a good sample as it is may be colonized w/ bacteria).
  - ○ **Abscess:** the wall of the cavity & NOT the pus (which is WBC & debris & may NOT have bacteria growing).
  - ○ **Osteomyelitis:** Cx curettage from the ulcer base following superficial debridement of necrotic tissue. Organisms cultured from superficial swabs are NOT reliable for predicting the pathogens responsible for deeper infx. Bone biopsy & Cx is important before Abx (especially in chronic osteo)

> **Attention:** Findings that indicate abx are failing (need to switch abx for possible resistance) → persistent fever after 48-72 hrs, clinical deterioration, worsening erythema (like for cellulitis if it's pen marked)

- **MRSA abx:** Vancomycin, Daptomycin & Linezolid (for hospital acquired MRSA) & Doxcycyline, Bactrim, Rifampin & Clinamycin (for community acquired MRSA).

Pseudomonas abx: Zosyn, cipro/Levofloxacin, Cefepime, Ceftazidime, Mero/Imi/Doripenem (Ertapenem is NOT good for Pseudomonas), Topramycin/Gyntamycin/Amikacine, Aztreonam, Fasfamycin, & Colistin

- **Same bioavailability if they are given IV or PO:** Azithromycin, Levofloxacin, Ciprofloxacin, doxycycline, clindamycin, linezolid, & fluconazole.
- **You can choose either IV or PO abx** depending on the specific infx you are treating. Endocarditis may need IV abx for 6 weeks (PICC line will be useful) but treating something like PNA or UTI→ it's ok to start IV & switch to PO or even begin w/ PO. PO intolerance makes IV rout a good option. For bacteremia start IV & check for one negative blood Cx. After 2-3 days switch to PO if negative.
- **Antimicrobial stewardship program** (program for wise abx use) De-escalation of therapy, IV to PO conversions, Dose optimization, Guidelines & clinical pathways, Education (Colonization vs. infx). Implementation of an antimicrobial stewardship program helps: Improve pt outcomes, Improve pt safety, Reduces resistance, & Reduces cost

15. Clostridium difficile infection (CDI)

C. difficile infx is a major cause of in pt gastrointestinal illness. C. difficile is a gram-positive, spore-forming, normal flora of the GI tract mostly spread by the fecal-PO route. Soap & water is the best for prophylaxis (alcohol foam does NOT eliminate spores).

Risk factors
Recent abx use is the main culprit, especially clindamycin, cephalosporins, & fluoroquinolones. Though, any abx can predispose to *C. difficile* overgrowth, including Vanc & metronidazole. Nursing home pts, elderly, immunosuppressed, & pts w/ altered GI anatomy (e.g., ileostomy, colostomy) are at ↑ risk.

Clinical features
Typical presentation is profuse watery diarrhea, lower abdominal pain/tenderness, & often extremely foul-smelling stool (nurses usually suspect that first).

Laboratory tests
The most accurate test is stool *C. difficile* antigen PCR. The disadvantage is that it takes around 24-48 hrs to return from the lab. Get CBC & CMP to assess severity.

Classification
Used to decide on Tx options, including possible ICU care.
- **Mild:** Diarrhea is the sole Sx.
- **Moderate:** Diarrhea plus additional signs & Sx NOT meeting criteria for severe or complicated CDI.
- **Severe:** Hypoalbuminemia (albumin <3), a WBC count >15 k, & abdominal tenderness. **Complicated CDI pts who need to be considered for ICU:** HoTN w/ or w/o vasopressors, fever > 38. 5°C, ileus, abdominal

distension, mental status changes, WBC count >35, 000or <2, 000, serum lactate level >2. 2 mmol/L, & any signs of end-organ failure.

Tx

Can be initiated before laboratory confirmation for pts w/ a ↑ pre-test suspicion. The offending abx should be stopped. If abx must be continued, treat w/ abx less known for causing CDI, such as aminoglycosides, macrolides, Vanc, or tetracycline.

- **For mild-to-moderate CDI**: PO metronidazole 500mg TID x10 days should be used. If the pt fails to respond to metronidazole therapy, a change in therapy to PO Vanc should be considered.
- **Severe or complicated disease:**
  w/o ileus → PO Vanc is administered (in addition to IV metronidazole)
  w/ ileus →Vanc delivered PO & per rectum plus IV metronidazole is to be given. Additionally, supportive care w/ fluid resuscitation, electrolyte replacement, & DVT prophylaxis should be continued. A CT abdomen & pelvis is recommended in pts w/ complicated CDI, as is a surgical consult due to possible need for subtotal colectomy & ileostomy, which is associated w/ ↓ mortality.
- **Recurrent disease:** The **first recurrence** of CDI should be treated w/ the same regimen used for the initial episode. However, if infx is severe, PO Vanc should be used. The **second recurrence** should be treated w/ Vanc PO. For a **third recurrence** after a pulsed Vanc regimen, fecal microbiota transplant (FMT) should be considered.

Special considerations

- **Fidaxomicin** was approved for mild-to-moderate CDI & was non-inferior to Vanc in phase III trials & **Fecal microbiol transplant (FMT**) has shown promising results in trials for recurrent CDI as mentioned above.

> **Attention:** Probiotics are NOT recommended according to current guidelines, especially in immunosuppressed pts, where there are a few case reports of bacteremia resulting from their use.

- **PO Vanc is expensive** but PO metronidazole is cheap.
- **Do NOT test C. diff in pts w/o diarrhea** (unless you have another reason like leukocytosis w/o known source). Monitor response to Tx by decreasing bowel movement numbers per day. Recovery is monitored clinically (usually no need to test negative C. diff as it can be positive after the Tx for months w/o the need to repeat abx & it is NOT a sign of Tx failure).
- **Start counting 14 days of anti C diff abx (like Flagyl or Vanc) from the time you stop the offending agent** (like Clindamycin). Do NOT undertreat in order to avoid recurrence.

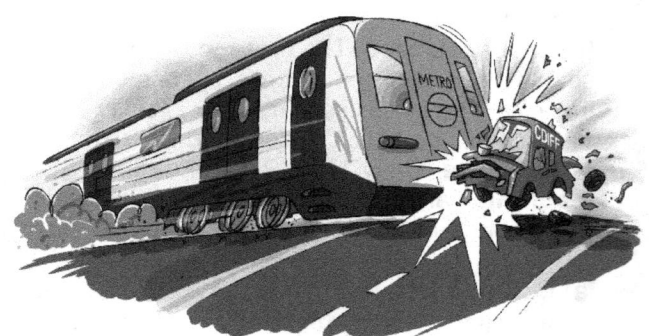

METROnidazole is effective against C diff infx.

16. Methicillin-Resistant Staphylococcus Aureus (MRSA)

Thisis a major cause of morbidity & mortality in hospitals. It can cause PNA, bacteremia & skin & skin structure infx (SSSIs). Tx has become challenging because of resistance & limited availability of antimicrobial agents. Moreover, there has been an emergence of community-acquired strains (CA-MRSA), which sometimes have a higher virulence than hospital-acquired ones.

Community-acquired MRSA

Clindamycin, trimethoprim-sulfamethoxazole (TMP-SMX) & tetracyclines (doxycycline) are recommended as first line agents for CA-MRSA, but should NOT be used for hospital-acquired strains due to ↑ resistance. Out of the 3 agents mentioned above, only clindamycin has good activity against both MRSA & beta-hemolytic Streptococci. Usually, in skin infx thought to be due to MRSA, empiric coverage for both MRSA & Streptococci is needed. However, using clindamycin as a sole agent can lead to resistance. Hence, TMP-SMX or doxycycline in combination w/ a beta-lactam agent, such as ampicillin or amoxicillin, is preferred.

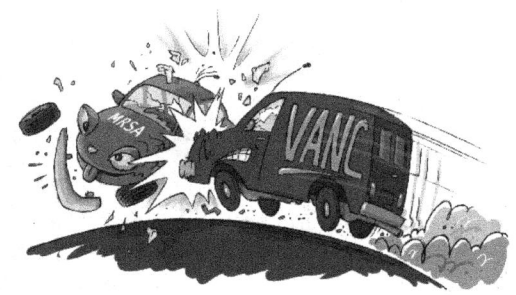

*VANcomycin is the 1st empiric IV Tx of choice for **MRSA**; especially for in pt.*

> **Attention**: Clindamycin is associated w/ a relatively higher risk for *c diff infx*.

Hospital-acquired MRSA: Nursing homes, dialysis centers, or any long-term healthcare facility. Has been treated w/ IV **Vanc** for several years. It is cheap, effective, & has years of experience behind its use as a first line agent. However, in recent years, there have been reports of ↑ resistance & rising minimum inhibitory concentrations (MICs).

There are several reports of emergence of VRSA (Vanc resistant *S. aureus*), VISA (Vanc intermediate *S. aureus*), & HVRSA (heterogeneous Vanc resistant *S. aureus*). However, as of now, it is still used as a first line agent for MRSA.
Vanc is a bactericidal agent & acts by inhibiting cell wall synthesis. It is used only in IV formulation (unless specifically treating *C. difficile* infx), & requires dose adjustment in renal insufficiency. Nephrotoxicity & red man syndrome are among the most common adverse effects associated w/ it, & require stopping the drug. Trough (blood level) should be checked regularly to assure therapeutic levels (make sure it is a true trough by checking it just before the next dose or before HD)**.**

Linezolid is another agent that can be used in both PO & IV formulations. It has good lung penetration & is recommended for MRSA PNA NOT responding well to Vanc & in pts being discharged back to a nursing home on PO meds.

Daptomycin is among the newer agents approved for Tx of MRSA. It is used for MRSA bacteremia, but is NOT recommended for use in MRSA PNA as it is inactivated by pulm surfactant. Additionally, it can be used for complicated skin infx & infective endocarditis. Adverse effects include myopathy (monitor CPK), peripheral neuropathy, & eosinophilic PNA.

Ceftaroline (Cephalosporins) is good for MRSA & is approved for PNA & cellulitis infx (NOT the 1st line though)

17. Acute kidney injury (AKI)/Chronic Kidney Disease (CKD)/End stage Renal Disease (ESRD)

AKI:

General: most common practical definition is an acute ↑ in serum Cr >0.3 from baseline (so it can occur in normal kidneys & impaired kidneys like CKD). Prerenal & postrenal causes should be distinguished from intrinsic renal parenchymal disease because they are rapidly reversible. Also divided into oliguric (<400 ml/24hr) & nonoliguric (>400 ml/24hr). The lower the urine output, the worse the prognosis.

Work up for AKI:

- Check **dehydration**, ↓ oral intake, HoTN (infx/sepsis in general) or bleeding as prerenal is very common cause for AKI & it is easy reversible by IV/PO fluid. Prevent expensive work up by good chart review & history.
- Check **new meds**, which maybe are NOT kidney friendly like ACEi/ NSAIDs & stop them/ monitor improvement (may NOT need further testing).
- **Urine analysis (UA)** to check for UTI, urine protein, blood, etc. Urine sediment examination for casts, cells & crystals are best done by Nephrology. The presence of WBC casts & Eosinophils in the urine may indicate Acute Interstitial Nephritis AIN (a type of intrinsic AKI usually caused by Beta-Lactam Abx). RBC casts are highly suggestive of glomerular pathology.
- **Kidney US** if you suspect postrenal (look for obstruction/hydronephrosis). Relief obstructions ASAP w/ either foley cath (if BPH) or nephrostomy (for maybe uretral stricture or

stones) depends on the level of the obstruction. Anuria or oliguria is maybe a clue (consider foley cath or bladder scan first before formal abdominalUS; cheaper/faster)

- **FeNa** can differentiate prerenal from intrinsic (like Acute Tubular necrosis ATN) AKI in pts w/ oliguria (although it is also commonly used w/ nonoliguric pts but has lower sensitivity). ↓ FeNa tells you that the kidney is "working" & keeping or reabsorbing most of the filtered Na to the blood, so the AKI can be treated w/ fluid because it is due to a prerenal etiology. If the pt is on diuretics, check FeUrea instead of FeNa (diuretics impair renal ability to reabsorb Na & give false values). FeNa can be calculated online by the values of both urine & serum Cr & Na.

> **Attention to** AKI from CHF exacerbation also could cause low FeNa but should NOT be given IVF

- Consider **peripheral blood smear** to check for schistocytes when there is suspicion for HUS, TTP, malignant HTN, or scleroderma renal crisis.
- **Look for signs of cirrhosis in pts w/ evidence of chronic liver disease or BNP/CXR in pts w/ CHF** as they both have ↓ effective intravascular volume perfusing the kidneys even though pts usually are volume overloaded. Cardiorenal & hepatorenal syndrome are hard to treat.

Management:
- **Start IV normal saline** for pts w/ volume depletion.
- **You can try albumin** for those w/ cirrhosis & intravascular volume depletion.

- **Review meds:** stop ACE inhibitor, diuretics, NSAIDs & any nephrotoxic meds
- **In case there is urinary obstruction:** place urinary cath to relieve bladder outlet obstruction. If the obstruction is above the bladder, consult urology for nephrostomy placement.
- **Monitor daily Cr & electrolytes** especially K, & daily ins/outs. Assess daily need for dialysis & signs of renal recovery.

CKD:

CKD is characterized by abnormality of kidney function (hematuria, proteinuria, etc) or an alternation in kidney function for > 3 months (elevated serum Cr & ↓ eGFR as above). Always compare Cr level to baseline values. Elevated Cr is a good indicator for impaired renal function but always calculate eGFR as it is takes into consideration other factors like: pt's age, sex & race. As Cr is a muscle product, ↓ body muscle mass (in thin pts) can give a falsely normal or low [Cr] even in the presence of CKD.

Stage	GFR
1*	≥90
2*	60–89
3a	45-59
3b	30-45
4	15–29 (needs preparation for kidney replacement therapy, dialysis)
5	<15 or on dialysis

*Need to have anatomical or functional renal abnormalities.

Attention: DM & HTN are common etiologies for CKD.

Common Etiologies:

- **Diabetic kidney disease:** Look for microalbuminuria, followed by proteinuria & declining GFR. The presence of retinopathy strongly suggests coexisting nephropathy.
- **Glomerular disease:** Look for glomerular hematuria, proteinuria, & HTN; if w/ systemic manifestations, lupus nephritis & postinfectious GN. If nephrotic syndrome is present look for FSGS, membranous nephropathy, minimal change disease & amyloidosis. Kidney biopsy is often needed to make the diagnosis.
- **Tubulointerstitial disease:** look for proteinuria, glycosuria, pyuria & leukocyte casts, as well as, papillary necrosis on ultrasound.
- **Structural disease**: like autosomal dominant polycystic kidney disease (ADPKD): HTN, hematuria & family hx of CKD.

Management:

- **Begin restriction** of Na (<2g/day if comorbid CHF or refractory HTN), Low K (60mEq/day), & low phosphorus (800-100mg/day) diet might be needed in patients with more advance CKD.
- **For HTN:** use ACE-I or ARBs, diuretics are commonly needed (use loop diuretics rather than thiazide for GFR<30)
- **For persistent microalbuminuria:** start ACE-I or ARBs even if pt is normotensive (for the kidney protection effect).
- **Anemia:** erythropoietin to maintain Hg between (10-11) & iron to maintain iron stores. Always check iron levels before stating erythropoietin as iron deficiency can coexist w/ anemia of chronic disease from CKD. Correct iron deficiency before starting erythropoietin.
- **Hypocalcaemia & Hyperphosphatemia:** Can lead to secondary hyperparathyroidism

manifested by & elevated Parathyroid hormone (PTH).

    1. Low phosphorus diet.

    2. Correcting Hyperphosphatemia – Use Ca based binders including: Ca Carbonate & Ca Acetate. Non-Ca based alternatives like Sevelamer

- **Metabolic acidosis:** Bicarb HCO_3 therapy to maintain HCO_3 between (20-26). Usually 650-1300mg TID.
- **Vitamin D deficiency:** CKD leads to ↓ production of calcitriol, which is the active form of Vit D. This also causes ↑ of PTH. Can give calcitriol once 25-OH Vit D repleted.

Special considerations:

- **Refer CKD to nephrologist in stage ≥3** for cause identification, complication management & timely preparation for transplant or dialysis (as AV fistula/graft needs weeks to months to maturate & be ready to be used). Avoid frequent BP measurements & unnecessary PICC/central line in such pts to save those peripheral & central veins for future possible HD life-saving accesses (consult nephrology in non-urgent cases for further recommendation)
- **Kidney transplant:** is associated w/ superior quality of life & is less expensive compared w/ long-term dialysis. All pts w/ ESRD are considered candidates for kidney transplant unless they have systemic malignancy, chronic infx, severe cardiovascular disease, or neuropsychiatric disorders. Transplantation is particularly beneficial in young pts.
- **Hemodialysis HD indication**: 1-refractory hyperkalemia (NOT responding to Kayexalate, insulin/dextrose, albuterol & lasix), acidemia (NOT responding to HCO_3 PO or IV), or volume overload (NOT responding to lasix or other loop

diuretics). 2-Signs & Sx of uremia (AMS, asterixis, pericardial friction rub, vomiting).

- **ESRD pts on HD**: usually get 3 session of HD a week. Compliance w/ HD, fluid restriction & ↓ Na/K/phosphate diet should be assessed regularly & monitoring body weight (for fluid overload) can be very informative. Pulm edema/congestion/CHF exacerbation may occur very often in non-compliant pts which necessitates urgent HD.
- **FE (Na) interpretation in pts w/ oliguria:** If >1% consider tubular damage such as ATN. If <1% & UA is normal, consider prerenal azotemia
- **ACEi is expected to** ↑ **Cr** as it lowers the intraglomerular pressure from vasodilatation on both afferent & efferent arterioles but more on efferent arterioles. This ↑ is NOT considered an AKI unless it is > 30% from baseline (so repeat Cr 2 weeks after ACEi initiation). Stop ACEi in such case & any case of AKI to avoid further compromising of renal perfusion.
- **Adjust medication doses according to eGFR** to prevent toxicity, especially meds cleared renally. Meds stay in the system longer in the case of AKI/CKD. (e.g. cause AMS in case of morphines & benzos & bleeding in case of novel anticoagx).

18. Volume Overload

A diagnosis of overloaded volume status can be elicited by a good h & p. It can be attributed to CHF (systolic mostly but also diastolic w/ preserved EF), cirrhosis, or nephropathy in most cases. In the in pt setting, volume overload is often iatrogenic caused simply by too much IV fluid or over-resuscitated truly hypovolemic pts (failure to adjust fluid infusion rate from replacement fluid deficit to maintenance rate). Often it is hard to assess volume status accurately.

History:

- **Ask about compliance w/ fluid restriction (1-1. 5 Liter) & ↓ Na⁺ diet,** especially for CHF pts. Any Na rich food & processed foods, salty foods may NOT necessarily taste salty to the pt. This is especially common during or around the holidays (eating at restaurants, canned foods, fried foods, etc).
- **Ask about meds compliance:** Have they skipped any doses of meds recently? Ask this question particularly to pts on diuretics who have complained about ↑ urinary frequency as a side effect. Also ask if they have been adjusting their Lasix or diuretic dose depending on their daily weight (Do they have scale at home)?
- **Have they taken or been prescribed any new meds recently?** One common culprit is NSAIDs (associated w/ worsening heart failure/HTN & of course worsening CKD).
- **Ask about missing dialysis** it is a common cause for volume overload & SOB/pulm edema hospital admissions. Always ask about recent weight change.

Exam & tests:

- Pts w/ volume status issues should be examined multiple times per day to assess the rate of diuresis or IV fluid infusion in case of hypo or hypervolemia (stop when pt is euvolemic).

- **Vitals:** especially BP (HoTN indicates poor LV function while elevated BP maybe the reason for diastolic or systolic CHF exacerbation).
- **Inspection**: ↑ daily weight, pitting edema which must be assessed over a bony surface such as the shins or metatarsals, pronounced neck veins & elevated JVP (↑ Sen. & Spec.) & be on the alert for IV fluids hanging in the pt's room that are flowing continuously when in fact these fluids should have been held. Dependent edema is commonly seen in bedridden or supine pts in flank regions.
- **Auscultation**: Crackles & rales, shifting dullness from ascites, high liver span assessed via percussion, S3 heart sound due to turbulent blood flow from high volume (gallop)
- **CXR**: to establish a baseline w/ serial x-rays to assess improvement in the case of pulm edema (CXR changes occur quickly in comparison to PNA infiltrations). Remember to look at the CXR yourself to assess for Kerley B lines, hilar haze, cephalization of pulm vasculature, thickening of pleural fissures, peribronchial cuffing, diffuse opacification (AKA complete white out), & pleural effusion.
- **TTE**: should be considered up front to evaluate & compare ejection fraction or at least establish a baseline.
- **RUQ ultrasound**: to evaluate for hepatomegaly & congestion.
- **Labs:** Serum Cr (elevated Cr usually indicates renal involvement which could be either AKI or ESRD w/ missed HD) & BNP (elevated BNP indicates volume overload).

Management:
For all pts: stop IV fluids & consider mnemonic LMNOP (Lasix, Morphine, nitrates, O_2, posture), which is basically Tx for pulm edema (pt is sick & needs emergent Tx). Also, recommend a ↓Na diet, fluid restriction, record daily ins & outs, encourage strict meds & HD compliance (if applicable).
For ESRD pts who have missed HD, arrange for dialysis, consult nephrology, & educate regarding compliance.
For cirrhosis pts w/ ascites, assess the need for therapeutic paracentesis & replace albumin (25 ml of albumin for every 2 liters of ascitic fluid removed).

Special considerations:

- **Pulmonary edema or congestion can occur w/o signs of peripheral edema** (lower extremities swelling, JVD, & hepatojugular reflex), especially if the etiology is HTN urgency/emergency w/ CHF & vice versa, peripheral edema can occur w/o pulm edema. The cornerstone of Tx is diuresis, especially for peripheral edema as these pts may sometimes have 10-20 liters of extra volume that needs to be eliminated.

> **Attention:** Pts w/ pulm edema from uncontrolled HTN w/o peripheral edema can be euvolumic (or even volume depleted from chronic diuresis) & diuresis should be brief along w/ controlling BP.

- **The physical examination** of pts who are volume depleted is often less telling than that of their overloaded counterparts.
- **Diuresis should be targeted** to achieve daily negative fluid balance. Net negative of 0.5-1L is usually safe, & might need to be more when

patient is symptomatic. Always check BMP (for K & Cr), Mg, & phosphate, & correct electrolyte abnormality as needed (Q 12 hrs). It is highly recommended to supplement K^+ & Mg^{2+} orally in the case of a high diuresis target, even if they are normal (prophylactically).

- **Usually loop diuresis w/ Lasix or Bumex either orally or IV** (PO meds do NOT absorb effectively due to intestinal edema in volume overload pts) is adequate. If the response is suboptimal, you can add thiazide diuretics like metolazone (once a day 30 minutes before the loop diuretic dose) for a synergetic effect.
- **Monitor serum Cr closely** as risk of AKI is a common consequence of overdiuresis. ↓diuretic dose (or even stop it) in case of Cr elevation (↓ urine output is another indicator for volume depletion). ↓central venous pressure (CVP) in ICU pts w/ a central line (normal CVP is 8-12) is a good sign of volume depletion (low CVP is almost always a sign of low volume status & indicating need for IV fluid).

> **Attention**: measure CVP "by yourself" as it is an essential value and you need it to be accurate.

- **NOT all edema or ascites needs diuresis** such as in the case of cirrhosis or malnutrition. In these cases, low oncotic pressure intravascularly causes "leakage" of the fluid into the interstitial space (third space). Pt's intravascular volume might be low & diuretics may NOT help. Measure CVP (if central line is available in the ICU) & urine Na. You may need to give IV fluid in the case of persistent low BP, ↓ CVP, ↓ urine Na^+ & signs of poor end organ perfusion, such as AKI. Improving nutrition may ↓ the edema (albumin infusion is expensive & does NOT help due to the short half life).

19. Volume Depletion

Most cases of volume depletion can be attributed to an etiology of gastrointestinal losses, renal losses, skin losses, third space sequestration, or iatrogenic causes.

H & P:

- GI loss like diarrhea or vomiting? GI bleeding indicated by either BRBPR or black, tarry stool? ↓ PO fluid intake for any reason such as an elderly pt w/ AMS, NPO w/o IV fluid, or excessive sweating? Finally: consider pancreatitis, trauma such as crush injuries (Which could reveal pancreatic injury), recent surgery, or abdominal pain that could indicate peritonitis. All of these etiologies could contribute to third spacing.

- **Vitals→** tachycardia (first sign usually but maybe masked by AV node blocking agents) & HoTN. Tachypnea for any reason can ↑ insatiable water loss & cause volume depletion.

- Helpful equations to know:
  MAP=CO x TPR
  CO= HR x SV
  MAP= HR x SV x TPR
  HR= MAP/SV x TPR.

  (Mean artery pressure MAP, Cardiac output CO, Total peripheral resistance TPR, Heart rate HR, Stroke volume SV).

- **Inspection:** malaise, fatigue, thirst, muscle cramping, syncope, postural dizziness, abdominal & CP due to ischemia of the mesenteric or coronary vasculature, confusion, & altered mental status due to ↓ cerebral vascular perfusion. Assess skin turgor or lack thereof & delayed capillary refill. Tachypnea may be present due to acidosis. Muscular irritability (or cramps) & confusion may be present due to metabolic alkalosis. Muscle weakness & cramping may be observed due to hyperkalemia or hypokalemia. Seizures & coma may occur due to hyponatremia or hypernatremia. Flattened neck veins may be noted.

- **Auscultation**➔Listen for groaning & moaning due to abdominal pain or CP as well as muscle cramping. Pts may tell you that they have been urinating more or even less frequently (due to AKI/ dehydration). Tachycardia & tachypnea may be present as mentioned above.
- **Labs: Check BMP** (elevated Cr usually indicates overdiuresis & intravascular volume depletion). Check **urine electrolytes** (urine Na & urine Cr along w/ BMP) & calculate **FeNa** (calculator **available online**) or **FeUrea** if pt is on diuresis (get urine Cr & urine Urea along w/ BMP). Calculate the **BUN to Cr ratio** (high in dehydration). Check **lactic acid** level to assess for lactic acidosis (usually q4-6hrs until resolution).

Management: IV hydration (mostly normal saline): start w/ few liters boluses (as needed) & then keep maintenance fluid (if can NOT tolerate PO).

Attention:
1. **Dehydration is different than hypovolemia** although they are treated mostly the same. Hypovolemia "low blood volume", which is NOT identical to dehydration "loss of water" because blood is NOT pure water.
2. **FeNa (&even FeUrea)** are very helpful to diagnose the etiology of **oliguria**. FeNa <1% ➔ prerenal (Tx mostly w/ hydration) vs >1➔renal/post-renal. FeNa is NOT very helpful in case of normal UOP.

---

20. Diabetes mellitus (DM)

Diabetes Mellitus (DM) is a common metabolic disturbance seen in U. S adults & occurs due to a defect in insulin secretion, action, or both. Around 11% of the U. S population >20 years old is affected. Around 90% of those cases belong to the type II category.

Classification: The majority of cases can be classified into one of two categories: type I (<10%) & type II (>90%). Other specific types of DM exist related to certain genetic defects, drugs, endocrinopathies, & other syndromes. Also, DM related to pregnancy is known as gestational diabetes mellitus (resolved after delivery, recurrent in subsequent gestations, & can become overt DM).

Diagnosis: suggested by any of the following criteria:
1. Plasma glucose > 126 mg/dl after an overnight fast (should be confirmed w/ a repeat test). Fasting glucose level between 100-125 mg/dl indicates Impaired Fasting Glucose (IFG).
2. Random glucose level > 200 mg/dl plus Sx of diabetes mellitus (polyuria, polydipsia, fatigue, weight loss). Values of 140-199 mg/dl indicate Impaired Glucose Tolerance (IGT).
3. PO glucose tolerance test, which shows a glucose level > 200 mg/dl 2 hrs after administration of a 75 gm glucose load.
4. HgbA1c>6. 5% (needs to be confirmed w/ any of the above).

Management: Glycemic control & management of other atherosclerosis risk factors like HTN (JNC-8 guidelines, target has changed to BP <140/90), HLD (LDL goal is <100 mg/dl), smoking, & monitor for diabetic end organ damage such as retinopathy & glomerulopathy (by early referral to ophthalmology, w/ in 10 years for type I & on the time of diagnoses for type II, & referral to nephrology in CKD stage III). Fasting CBG should be between 70 to 130 mg/dl & postprandial CBG should be targeted to <180 mg/dl w/ Hgb A1c < 7%. For in pt (especially critically ill pts) target CBG should NOT be strictly controlled → okay <180 to avoid hypoglycemia. Consider more strict A1c control (<5.5%) in CF & pregnant pts.

DM Type I: Type I requires lifelong insulin replacement. The sooner DM II is diagnosed, the more insulin secreting beta cells will be saved from destruction & the easier DM will be managed.

Type of insulin	Onset of action (hrs)	Peak effect (hrs)	Effect duration (hrs)
Rapid acting			
Lispro/Aspart/Glulisi-ne	<15min	≈1	3-5
Regular (draw 1st in syringe if mixed w/ NPH)	≈1	2-4	6-8
Intermediate acting			
NPH (only one cloudy, rest clear)	≈1.5	6-8	12-16
Long acting			
Glargine	1-2	0	Up to 24
Levemir/Detemir	1-2	0	Up to 24

Usually, in an average pt, total daily dose (TDD) of insulin is calculated by the following formula: 0.2-0.8 units/kg per day (0. 2 units/kg is usually started in a newly diagnosed/insulin naive pt). About 50% of the dose is usually basal insulin (intermediate or long-acting insulin, either NPH twice daily or detemir/glargine once daily), & the rest can be divided to three times/day before meals (or even twice depending on the compliance).

Two of the most commonly used regimens are:

1. **NPH & regular (2-3 injections/day):** Calculate Total Daily Dose TDD as per 0.4-0.8 units/kg. Divide it ½ & ½ OR 2/3rd & 1/3rd in morning & evening, depending on the biggest meal in the day. Divide the morning dose administered w/ breakfast into 2/3rd NPH & 1/3rd regular.

   Divide the evening dose into ½ NPH (to be administered at bedtime) & ½ regular (to be administered w/ evening meal). Then, calculate the correction factor by the following formula: 1700 divided by the TDD.
   This means that 1 unit of insulin will bring down the glucose by approximately x mg (x-correction factor, try to make the numbers easy to calculate like 50, 60, etc.). **Correction factor calculation is time consuming & can be avoided safely most of the time.**

   This regimen is also the cheapest available on the market. It is a good regimen for non-insured, newly diagnosed DM, & non-compliant pts as it needs fewer sticks.
   NPH & regular insulin can be prescribed also as a pre-mixed combination of 70% NPH/30% regular regimen (commonly known as 70/30) & it can be given twice daily (before breakfast & lunch or lunch & dinner, depends on the two largest meals)

2. **Glargine & aspart/lispro/regular (four times a day regimen):** Usually 50% of TDD is administered as long-acting glargine at night, & the remaining dose is divided into 3 times a day as rapid acting insulin given w/ meals.

   Supplemental sliding scale SSS can be added to the scheduled doses for better DM control (increase the scheduled insulin dose according to the previous day requirement from the SSS).

CBGs should be monitored both as an in pt & as an out pt at least 3-4 times/day (2 times is acceptable for out pt). Monitoring should include fasting CBG pre-breakfast & random post-prandial checks (writing them in a log can help in adjusting insulin doses).

Type II DM: Initial therapy is w/ PO agents. **Metformin** is commonly used as it has an added benefit of reducing obesity ($\downarrow$ mortality as well). Also, it does NOT cause hypoglycemia (adverse reactions: N/V, & diarrhea). However, it should be used w/ caution in pts w/ renal disease (avoid in CKDIII or more as it could cause lactic acidosis). Sulfonylureas (SFU) such as glipizide, glyburide, & glimepiride are also used commonly.

Other non-SFU analogues such as nateglinide & repaglinide are rarely used. Other options include alpha-glucosidase inhibitor acarbose, thiazolidinediones such as rosiglitazone or pioglitazone (can cause fluid retention & should thus be used w/ caution in cardiac or renal disease), dipeptidyl peptidase-4 inhibitors sitagliptin & saxagliptin, bile acid sequestrant colesevelam, & glucagon-like peptide agonists such as exenatide. Eventually, type II DM pts end up needing insulin, which should be started as discussed above.

Diabetic ketoacidosis:
DKA occurs in up to 5% of pts w/ type I DM & can rarely occur in type II DM as well. It is often precipitated due to interruption of insulin dose when the pt feels sick. Precipitating factors could be a UTI, PNA, sepsis, MI, or trauma.
Usually include polyuria, polydipsia, N/V, abdominal pain, & signs of dehydration. Labs will show an elevated anion gap metabolic acidosis, elevated CBGs (however DKA can also rarely occur w/ normal CBGs), & electrolyte abnormalities.

Management:
Should include **fluid replacement therapy & insulin.**
Fluid replacement therapy is extremely important & should be started w/o delay. There is a fluid deficit of several liters, which should be replaced w/ normal saline boluses until vital signs stabilize & urine output is established.

After initial boluses, free water deficit is replaced w/ maintenance fluids (either normal saline or 0. 45% saline at 150–500 ml/hr for severe hypernatremia; always remember to correct Na for CBG).
Insulin therapy is usually started w/ initial fluid replacement. A bolus of regular insulin at 0.1 units/kg is given as soon as possible. Then, an insulin drip at 0.1 units/kg/hr is started. CBG should be lowered gradually at a rate of 50-75 mg/dl/hr (excess rapid correction>100 mg/dl/hr can lead to osmotic encephalopathy).

BMP & CBGs need to be monitored every 2 hrs.
Once CBG reaches 250 mg/dL, fluids should be changed to dextrose (5%) in 0. 45% saline to prevent dangerous hypoglycemia.

Insulin drip is continued until anion gap closes & pt has clinically improved. Subcutaneous insulin is usually started once pt starts eating. Always remember to continue the insulin drip for an hr after administration of subcutaneous insulin as it takes time to take effect.

Potassium: K deficit should always be anticipated, even if initial BMP shows normal K, as insulin administration can cause shift of K intracellularly. K should be routinely added to IV fluids at a rate of 10-20 meq/hr except in pts w/ hyperkalemia (>6 mmol/hr), renal failure, or oliguria. Bicarbonate, phosphate, & Mg rarely need to be replaced.

Bicarbonate: therapy in DKA is indicated only if pH <7. 1, shock/coma, plasma bicarbonate <5, acidosis-induced cardiorespiratory dysfunction, or severe hyperkalemia. When discharging pts w/ DKA, always remember to provide DM education to prevent further episodes.

Hyperosmolar non-ketotic syndrome (HONK):

Commonly seen in type II DM. It is very similar to DKA w/ some difference. HONK is typically more insidious in onset w/ dehydration (due to diuresis effect of the very high blood glucose) & some neurological deficits. No or mild ketoacidosis in HONK (PH >7.30 & HCO3 >15) compared to DKA (anion gab metabolic acidosis) due to the presence of insulin in the former (prevent lipolysis). **Tx:** same as DKA; especially **IV hydration**.

Hypoglycemia:

Common in the in pt setting & is often iatrogenic or caused by inadequate PO intake.

Management:

For conscious pts, orange juice, candy bars, fruits, & crackers can be given immediately (or Glucose tablets). IV dextrose should be used for pts w/ AMS. Initial bolus of 20 to 50 mL of 50% dextrose followed by an infusion D5W should be administered w/o delay.
Glucagon 1 mg IM/SC can be administered for those who are unable to take PO or who do NOT have IV access (or pts w/ "bad veins" & hard to get IV access on).

Complications of diabetes:

Long-term complications are divided into microvascular & macrovascular. Microvascular include diabetic retinopathy (usually the 1st one to occur), nephropathy, & neuropathy. Coronary artery disease & peripheral vascular disease are some of the macrovascular complications.

Attention: Tight CBG control (A1c <6.5-7%)→ reduce microvascular complications w/ minimal to no benefit for macrovascular complications (so pts w/ CVA, PAD or CAD may target A1c 7-8, especially w/ hx of hypoglycemia). Young pts → A1c <6.5-7%.

Routine screening: Pts w/ newly diagnosed type II DM should get an ophthalmology referral (yearly) to screen for diabetic retinopathy (possible laser Tx for non/proliferative retinopathy or "leaky vessels" to prevent blindness). For type I DM, it is usually recommended 5 years after diagnosis. Urine microalbumin (yearly), lipid panel, neurological exam & detailed foot exam should be done in yearly basis or more often (PRN).

Special considerations:

- **ACE inhibitors or ARBs are recommended** as 1st line for HTN w/ DM as they are known to prevent renal complications.
- **Standard insulin concentration is 100 units/mL (U-100).** Rarely, a highly concentrated form of insulin U-500 (500 units/mL) is used (when you need a very high dose of U-100 like 100s)
- **Diabetes mellitus in hospitalized pts:** Numerous studies have been done on glycemic control in hospitalized pts. The generally accepted target is 140 for floor pts & 180 for ICU pts (or critically ill pts). Avoidance of hypoglycemia should be a priority in both ICU & non-ICU pts.
- **In general: Insulin should be started for all DM type I & DM type II if oral meds failed** to control A1c (<6.5 - 7%). Consider starting insulin for DM type II if A1c is very high on the initial presentation (like >10%) due to the fact that oral

meds ↓ A1c around 1% per one med (usually you can NOT use more than 3 oral meds). Certain compliant pts can still control their A1c with diet, exercise & oral meds even if A1c is >10 on the presentation.

- **Supplemental insulin (less preferred term is sliding scale insulin):** is commonly used in addition to the scheduled dose for in pt to better control CBG. For optimal DM management, scheduled doses should be adjusted in a daily bases (at AM) according to the previous day supplemental insulin doses (if the pt expected to have the same calorie intake). So if pt is scheduled for 5 U aspart before dinner & he/she took 2 U after dinner on the supplemental scale → give 7 U aspart instead of 5 U the next evening.

- **Hypoglycemia:** usually when CBG <50-60.
  Sx: AMS (even coma) and/or sympathetic nervous system stimulation (palpitation, sweating, & anxiety).
  Etiology: diabetics w/ insulin over dosing, skipping meals, oral diabetes meds (especially in setting of AKI or CKD), sepsis, adrenal insufficiency, EtOH or exercise (w/o ↓ insulin dose).
  Management: check A1c, cortisol, TSH, UDS, possible infx, & C peptide (exogenous insulin?). Consider glucose tolerance test, review meds (especially new ones) & prediabetes (in DMII when insulin resistance ↑ →reactive hypoglycemia from ↑ insulin secretion after meals →Tx w/ metformin!). Tx w/ PO sugary fluid, IV dextrose (amp of D50% or drip D5/D10).

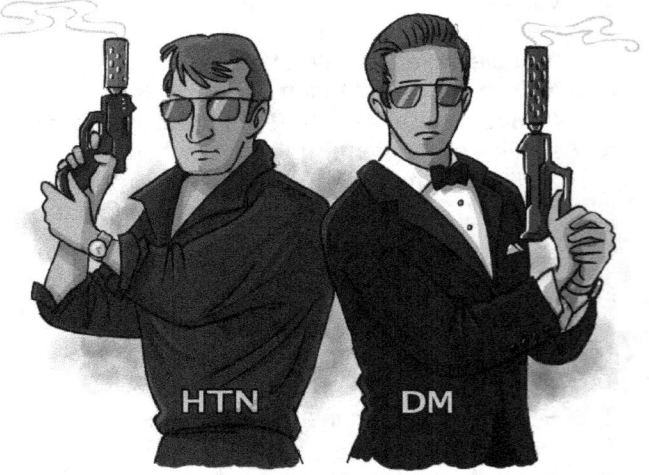

"THE SILENT KILLERS"

HTN & DM are the "silent killers" & may NOT cause symptoms. Treat & follow the numbers as appropriate.

21. Night float

This is a quick snap shot of the most common calls you may encounter while you are covering in pt nights. More comprehensive details are discussed in other sections.

Chest pain: **always examine the pt**. Consider in your differential diagnosis problems, which could be catastrophic to miss such as MI, pulm embolism/DVT, & pneumothorax. Do the appropriate exam & consider EKG, troponin, CXR, ABG (if there is dyspnea or desaturation on pulse Ox), O_2 mask, & D-dimer (discouraged to use for in pt).

> **Attention**: Consider heparin drip, ASA, NTG, morphine prn if NOT contraindicated according to your initial evaluation if you suspect ACS. Consider heparin drip also even before CTA if you highly suspect pulm embolism (immobility, tachypnea, tachycardia, & desaturation) & the rest of exam did NOT indicate otherwise.

Abdominal pain: **always examine the pt**. R/o surgical abdomen & other associated sx, which may indicate causes other than simple indigestion (like N/V, fever, diarrhea, diaphoresis & ↓ appetite). Consider EKG if high suspicion for inferior MI. Abdominal X-ray can show SBO (air/fluid levels), ileus (severely sick/opioids), fecal impaction (solid fecal material on the left abdomen). Consider PPI, Pepto-Bismol, pain meds as indicated & treat the underlying problem.

Fever: Consider CBC w/ diff, blood Cx, Urinalysis (UA) & urine Cx, CXR, & starting/adding/switching Abx. Examine the pt & see what is indicated. Usually if the fever is the only sign w/o cough, sputum, HA, nuchal rigidity, AMS, urinary Sx, abdominal pain, consider doing them all. Fever w/ AMS may need lumbar puncture (LP)

& /or CT scan of head w/ contrast (r/o meningitis especially if focal neuro deficits are present). If there is a known reason for fever like PNA or abscess & the pt is on the right abx, you can consider giving Tylenol (abx may need 1-2 days to fully work). That is unless the pt was afebrile for 24 hrs & then spiked a fever again; then you may need to send another set of cultures & possibly switch/add abx (may be resistant bug).

Insomnia: check sleep hygiene (avoid day napping, adequate daylight exposure, eating close to the sleeping time, caffeine intake, relaxing bedtime routine w/ less excessive night activities). Environmental changes like opening the curtains for light in the morning or sitting on bed or chair w/ physical therapy & early mobility in the morning may help. Use low dose benzos (like ambien or ativan) cautiously & temporarily especially in elderly (better to use mirtazapine or olanzapine/zolpidem) & it is better if you could avoid meds.

Critical electrolytes result:
- **Hypokalmia:** replaced by PO Kcl 10, 20, 40, 80 meq (tastes bad & could cause N/V & GI upset) or IV (called minibag) Kcl 10, 20 meq (dose 20 needs central line due to irritation, one bag usually takes 1-2 hrs). Usually each 10 meq PO or IV replaces 0. 1 of K in the blood. So if pt's K is 2. 8, give at least 70 to 100 meq (especially if you have hypokalemic-inducing factors like loop diuretics or vomiting). Check EKG (T wave flattening) & assess the route & urgency for K replacement. Keep it above 4 meq especially in CHF pts due to diuretic use.
- **Hyperkalemia:** give Kayexalate PO, which is a non-absorbable ion-exchange resin in GI system (it can be given by enema if NOT tolerating PO). Usually it takes hrs to work (can cause intestinal necrosis; avoid postoperatively & if constipation existed/ developed). You can give insulin & D5

fluids & Ca gluconate (stabilize the myocardium membrane & protect from arrhythmias) in case of EKG changes (T wave peaking). HD to ↓ K is always an option especially for pts already on HD. EKG changes → Ca gluconate + above options.

- **Hypocalcemia:** look at the albumin first & correct the Ca results (as the albumin carries the Ca & it can give pseudohypocalcemia in case of hypoalbuminemia). The correction factor is to add 0.8mg to the total Ca for each 1g drop in albumin. Normal low Ca is 8. 2 & normal low albumin is 3. 2, so if Ca is 7mg & albumin is 2g, no need to replace Ca. PO Ca is $CaCo_3$ & IV Ca is Ca gluconate (1-2 gr IV is the usual replacement dose). You can check ionized Ca for critical pts & no need for albumin correction in that case.
- **Hypophosphatemia:** PO form is Neutraphos & IV form is K-phos or Na-phos & dose is autocalculated.
- **Hypomagnesemia:** Mg oxide PO (comes as 400, 800mg) & Mg sulfate IV (dose is mostly autocalculated). Keep it above 2mg especially in CHF pts due to diuresis use. Milk of Magnesia (Mg hydroxide is a laxative)

Constipation: look for abdominal pain, abdominal distention, guarding (or any sign of surgical abdomen), N/V. Ask about PMH & meds which could cause constipation or ileus & electrolytes for hypercalcemia or hypokalemia which may cause constipation. If any of these alarming Sx are positive, proceed w/ treating underlying issue or call surgery if surgical abdomen presented (usually it is NOT surgical/ileus is NOT surgical). Digital rectal exam can be helpful to check for stool impaction (could be therapeutic as well). In general, if chronic, consider docusate, milk of magnesia, MiraLax (all PO). You can use water enema or Bisacodyl suppositories. If acute constipation, consider ruling out

SBO, volvulus, ileus, new opioid use w/o laxatives by ordering abdominal X-ray & if negative, proceed w/ as above.

A fib w/ RVR: always examine the pt, usually HR>110-120 & it needs an urgent action as the pt could develop tachycardia-related cardiomyopathy if left untreated even if asymptomatic. Check BP & ask about CP, feeling of palpitation, dizziness, blurry vision, & SOB. If any is present, consider urgent/emergent electric cardioversion. If not, try to slow the heart w/ : PO metoprolol, PO diltiazem, IV, metoprolol (10mg) bolus, IVdiltiazem bolus (20mg q15minute in general or 0.25mg/kg for low body weight), & IV amiodarone. Consider anticoagx according to CHADS2 score but it is NOT as urgent as controlling the rate. Consider MICU transfer if RVR is refractory to PO meds & IV boluses for IV continuous drip meds like diltiazem or amiodarone.

Headache HA: Tylenol is great for HA. Ask for the chronicity of the HA, acute onset is more concerning than chronic. R/o by hx, "the worst HA in my life" (SAH), focal neurological deficits by appropriate neuro exam (r/o CVA), fall/trauma (r/o Intracranial IC bleeding) & nuchal rigidity/fever (meningitis). Ask what meds the pt takes usually for his/her HA. Stress HA is a common type & responds to simple Tylenol. Consider CT scan if indicated.

Itching: Broad DDx (uremia, cirrhosis, idiopathic, etc). R/o allergic reaction, review meds & stop the new ones, which may be the culprit. Assess for anaphylactic Sx like SOB/tongue edema & respond as appropriate (IV epinephrine, IV Solu-Medrdol, IV Benadryl & consider intubation/ENT consult). Relieve w/ Benadryl or Atarax (PO or IV). Think about a more serious diagnosis when you see alarming signs like skin ulcers, rash, fever, boluses (dermatology consult for TSS or Steven Johnson Syndrome).

Nausea & vomiting: If these are new Sx, ask about other related Sx like abd. Pain, diarrhea, constipation, CP, fever or possible DKA picture & evaluate/treat as indicated. Symptomatic management w/ PO/IV Zofran, Phenergan & Reglan.

Fall: **always examine the pt,** ask about how it happened, where, witnesses, Coagx status, from how high, head trauma, LOC, N/V, focal neuro deficits, vision/pupils, & skeletal tenderness. If neuro exam is NOT changed from before, no LOC, no other signs of intracranial bleeding: neuro exam q1h for a few hrs afterwards by an MD or a nurse may be enough (although you can do CT scan w/o contrast if you have a high concern even w/ negative exam). Document your evaluation, order CT scan head, & bone x-rays, & prescribe pain meds as indicated.

Altered Mental Status (AMS): **always examine the pt,** broad DDx. In general, make sure vitals are stable, O_2 sat & CBG are okay, look for infx signs like UTI, PNA or bacteremia as indicated, check the admission diagnosis as it may be related to the AMS like fever in elderly. If your initial exam is normal, give PO/IV haldol, PO/IM Olanzapine (for elderly), PO/IV Ativan (avoid benzos for elderly). Consider wrist strains if they are at risk to harm themselves like pulling IV lines. Consider EtOH withdrawal & give PRN ativan (they may need high doses)

Hypo/hyperglycemia: Hypo is more serious than hyper due to neurological impairment, which can be caused by hypoglycemia especially for a long term. Check for sympathetic Sx like tachycardia, diaphoresis, AMS, & tremors for hypoglycemia. Give PO juice, cookies, 50cc D50 IV bolus (or called amp) or even IV D5 or D10 depending on responsiveness & Sx & ↓ insulin dose. Try NOT to hold long acting insulin (lantus or NPH) in case of corrected hypoglycemia episode. For hyperglycemia, calculate the correction factor (CF) & give fast acting insulin (regular or aspart), which is usually called supplemental or sliding scale.

Shortness of Breath/Hypoxia/Hypercapnia: always examine the pt. Broad DDx, usually comes together & the evaluation is usually similar. In general, think about pulm embolism ($\downarrow O_2 \downarrow CO_2$), pulm edema (excessive IV fluid/CHF), excessive respiratory secretions (deep suction resolves Sx quickly), worsening COPD/asthma/PNA (wheezing & consolidation), Pneumothorax (especially if they had recent lung procedure like thoracentesis/bronchoscopy/central line), recent blood transfusion in the last 24 hrs (Transfusion Related Acute Lung Injury (TRALI)). Consider O_2 masks, NIV (non-invasive ventilation, which is a tight mask to deliver more O_2), intubation, CXR, ABG, troponin, CBC, lactic acid, MICU consult, lasix, morphine as indicated (follow ACLS algorithm if pt is unstable).

Special consideration:
- **Call upper level in case of complicated picture** for second opinion.
- **Assess for the need for MICU transfer** in case of hemodynamic instability, hard to manage on the floor (due to need of intubation or IV drip for heart rate control in case of A fib w/ RVR for instance), need for q1hr CBG in case of refractory hypoglycemia, alcohol withdrawal Sx need a lot of Ativan (usually >10 mg in last 24h) or any other problem may need an ICU evaluation.
- **Giving too much O_2 in COPD pt causes respiratory depression (common mistake)** since respiratory drive is controlled by hypoxemia (normal person have the respiratory drive from hypercapnia which is NOT working for COPD pts due to chronic CO_2 retention). So a lot of O_2 is bad for COPD pts who retain CO_2 (O_2 sat between 88-92% is may be acceptable).

Chronic hypercapnia may NOT feel the sedation effect of CO_2 until $PaCO_2$ >90-100 while normally sedation is noted when $PaCO_2$ 60-70.

- **Mg, K, & Ca are connected & need to be corrected simultaneously:** Mg is needed in order for parathyroid gland to sense hypocalcemia & secrete PTH. The kidney tries to keep Mg in blood (in hypomagnesemia) & excrete K in urine in that process. That makes hypocalcemia & hypokalemia refractory to replacement if Mg is NOT corrected first.
- **Do EKG first** when you have K or Ca abnormality & correct faster in case of T wave changes.

23. Alarming findings

These following findings may indicate a serious diagnosis requiring fast action to prevent imminent morbidity & mortality or would indicate or require further management due to possible hidden serious disease.

- **GERD w/ dysphagia,** odynophagia, weight loss, anemia, GI bleed, long term GERD, & old age (>50) requires an upper endoscopy to r/o Barrett's esophagus & adenocarcinoma.
- **Neutropenia w/ fever** (>38.3 c) requires pan-cultures (to seek out the infx source), CXR (PNA), urine analysis (UTI), & empiric abx (Vanc, Zosyn, & possibly fluconazole).
- **Unexplained microcytic anemia** requires colonoscopy to r/o colon cancer.
- **Benign prostatic hypertrophy w/ back pain** requires back X-ray & PSA test due to suspicion of prostate cancer.
- **Known ulcerative colitis w/ abdominal pain & fever** high suspicion for toxic megacolon & requires an abdominal X-ray. You may also consider treating w/ ↑ dose IV steroids & consulting surgery.
- **Anorexia, cachexia, weight loss, & lymphadenopathy** are suspicious signs for cancer & age appropriate cancer screening should be done.
- **Change in stool caliber** may indicate distal colon cancer & should be alarming. Consider colonoscopy, especially if >50 years old or family hx of colon cancer (look for microcytic anemia for another clue).
- **Back pain w/** incontinence & saddle paresthesia indicates spinal cord compression. This requires a high dose IV steroid; radiotherapy & a surgery consult ASAP (make sure you get Biopsy mostly by IR to help in diagnoses if cancer is suspected).

- **HAs w/ temporal tenderness** may indicate Giant cell arteritis & it may requires high dose IV steroids. To prevent blindness, begin steroids before waiting for elevated ESR lab results.
- **CP w/ ST segment elevation** requires cards consult & cath lab (or thrombolytics depending on the facility) & giving urgent medicine in a short time frame (revascularization in <90 minutes). Urgent meds: ASA 325, plavix 600, Heparin drip, metoprolol (if SBP>100), NTG SQ, SL, IV (if NOT contraindicated), O_2 (if desating), morphine prn (if still in pain after NTG).
- **Asthma or COPD exacerbation pts who canNOT make a complete sentence** due to their SOB require immediate action. Administer O_2, jet nebs (Ventolin & ipratropium), & IV steroids. Consider a stat ICU evaluation while awaiting ABGs & CXR results if pt's Sx do NOT improve (for possible intubation).

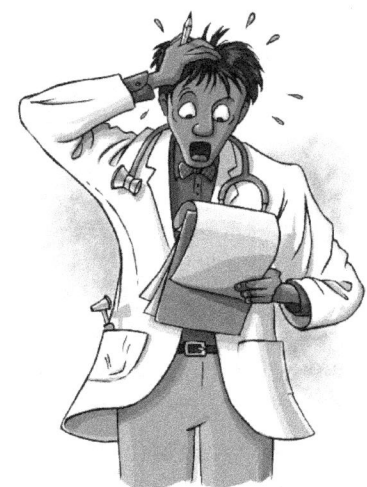

Some signs may be alarming for another serious condition; recognize those signs.

24. Home vs. floor vs. MICU triage

*Triage: in the simplest terms means the process of determining the priority of pts' Tx based on the severity of their condition. This section is mainly focused to help interns triage on crossover, night float, & in the ICU. The 1st level of triaging is done by the emergency physicians, so we have to become familiar w/ their classification. Therefore, when they call for an admission we know the level of acuity based on the **Emergency Severity Index (ESI)** from **1** which indicate **severe** case (may need intensive care) to **5** which indicate **mild** case (may be managed in an out pt setting)*

Example of ESI level 1: cardiac arrest, respiratory arrest, severe respiratory arrest, overdose w/ respiratory depression, hypoperfusion, anaphylactic shock, Symptomatic bradycardia, CP w/ hemodynamic instability.

Based on the ESI level 1 you know the pt will need a higher acuity of care, so these pts will go to the MICU, CCU, NICU, or a step down unit, if your hospital has one.

After the pt is triaged by the nursing staff, the pt is seen by the ER physician or resident, then medicine is called for evaluation of the pt either for admission, ICU placement, cardiology service, observation, or home.

> **Attention:** Always evaluate at the bedside in the ED & do NOT dismiss pts on the phone.

Based on lab values because labs might look ok, but the pt is not. See the pt, get a good H & P & use your clinical judgment. The emergency physicians are really busy, & they will NOT have the same time to get all the information.

If you feel the pt needs to be discharged, discuss w/ an upper level, fellow, or attending, then speak w/ the ER physician.

If the pt needs to go the ICU or cardiology service, justify your reasons & see if the ER physician will call Cardiology or MICU for evaluation before you admit. The ER physician's job is to provide acute care & send the pt to the proper service. Sometimes they need to get pts admitted fast to prevent ER boarding (overcrowding).

Special consideration:

- **Pneumonia:** good standard guide for admission is **CURB-65:** Confusion, Urea (BUN >20), Respiratory Rate >30, Blood pressure >90/60, Age >65. Score of 0-1: out pt, Score of 2: in pt wards, Score of 3 or greater: assess for ICU.
- **Diabetic ketoacidosis DKA: (**w/ elevated anion gap) needs ICU management (IV fluid, insulin, electrolytes control, etc) until the gap is closed & pt is switched from insulin drip to SQ when PO intake is tolerated.
- **Low systolic BP <90 w/ Sx (**make sure it is NOT chronic asymptomatic like in some dialysis pts) who are NOT responding to initial fluid challenge (like 1-2 Liter of NS), consider ICU evaluation for pressers use & close monitoring. Always know the vitals as most of the time your decision will be affected by them. Whoever you will discuss the pt w/ will want to know the vitals so he/she can forward their thinking.
- **Some interventions needs to be done in the ICU like:** IV β blocker or Ca blockers like metoprolol & diltiazem (for a fib & SVT), intubation & non-invasive ventilation, BP support infusion, arterial line placement for close BP monitoring, etc. Status post code-blue is a common ICU admission.

25. Cascade of actions for common problems

Common diagnosis or lab results abnormalities sometime should trigger a cascade of actions, which are like reflexes to those abnormalities. Memorizing those actions will minimize mistakes & save time in busy service. Following are some examples:

- **Electrolytes abnormalities:**
  Like hypernatremia for instance; should trigger
  1. Find the reason (like hypovolemia from ↓ PO intake)
  2. Intervene (like starting IV normal saline, encourage PO intake or start NJ tube/PEG tube free water flushes).

> **Attention:** to calculate how much fluid you are giving depends on the free water deficits (try to put the # of the liters you are giving in the order so you do NOT forget the fluid running)

  3. Follow up w/ your intervention: like schedule BMP q 4 hrs to make sure that you intervention is working & NOT over correcting or correcting too fast (if so, ↓ the rate of the fluid)
- **Hypothrombocytopenia:** ↓ in platelets more than 50% in 24 hrs after starting any type of heparin.
  1. Suspect HIT syndrome
  2. Stop heparin
  3. Send for HIT antibodies
  4. Start Argatroban (direct Xa factor inhibitor) & watch for thrombotic events (although there is ↓ platelets but w/ HIT syndrome there is ↑ risk for thrombosis)
  5. Ask nursing to NOT flush any IV line w/ heparin (write a note on the pt's door)

6. Stop Argatroban if HIT antibodies is negative
- **Chest pain:** consider EKG, troponin (q6 hrs for 3 times), CXR, ABG, O_2, heparin drip, NTG, morphine, CTA or cardiology consult. Choose what's appropriate depends on the exam to r/o critical conditions like ACS, pulmonary embolism & pneumothorax. Use you clinical judgment & do NOT overshot w/ all those previous intervention if ACS was just ruled out recently, clear other reason for CP like PNA, obvious chest tenderness w/ recent trauma or low suspicion for those conditions (young age w/ no comorbidities & psychiatric hx).
- **GI bleeding:**
  1. Check vitals including orthostatic BP
  2. Establish 2 large bore IV lines & start fluids resuscitation
  3. Start pantoprazole drip (in case the bleeding is from the stomach)
  4. Call GI for EGD or colonoscopy as appropriate
  5. Get CBC & schedule q4-6 hrs H & H to assess for ongoing bleeding
- **Fever (or any infectious sign):**
  1. Localize the infx site (cough/SOB→ PNA, urinary Sx→ UTI, chills/looking sick→ any infx including bacteremia, abdominal pain→ cholecystitis, appendicitis, diverticulitis or other abdominal infx)
  2. Send for culture as appropriate (send all cultures like urine, blood, sputum if no clear infx site)
  3. Get CBC w/ differentials to look for WBC & bands
  4. Start empirical abx (like Vanc & zosyn) as appropriate along w/ fluid IV
  5. Consider MICU evaluation for very sick pts (especially pts w/ ↑ SIRS score & shock pts w/ ↓ BP who did NOT response to 2-3 liters of IV NS)

6. Consider life-threatening infx like meningitis if you have AMS or physical exam finding suggesting it like HAs, neurological deficits or nuchal rigidity

7. Consider sliding scale insulin in addition to smaller than usual scheduled insulin dose: as infx will ↑ blood glucose but pt will have low appetite.

- **Unresponsiveness:** ACLS has the best algorithm to follow (**available online**). For pt w/ normal vitals but has ↓ level of consciousness:

  1. Check CBG (especially for diabetics on insulin) & give 50% dextrose amp if CBG is ↓.

  2. Check a recent medicine intake like morphine or benzodiazepines & give naloxone (you should see an immediate response if it is the reason for the AMS)

  3. Check urine drug screen as appropriate

  4. Consider CNS etiology like CVA or meningitis & get CT scan or lumbar puncture.

- **Death:**

  1. Check response to painful stimulas (sternal rub), **pulse** (check heart mintor, if available), **breathing sounds** (for like 1-2 minutes), **pupils reaction to light** at the bedside (& the general appearance like pale, cold & loss of muscle strength)

  2. Pronounce the death (military time) & offer condolences & empathy w/ the family

  3. Ask family when it is appropriate about organ donations (even if the pt is NOT qualified just for the paper work), autopsy to know the exact death reason; need to call the chaplain & if they need help in funeral home arrangement.

  4. Proceed w/ the paper work. You will need to list the most appropriate reason for death (like infx, sepsis, PNA, cancer, heart failure & so forth). Cardio respiratory failure by itself is NOT enough to be the only reason for death (as everybody die eventually from that reason).

- **Placement:** pts who are NOT able to live by themselves any more, for different reasons, will need placement plan early enough in order to ↓ length of hospital stay. Lack of family support, different chronic medical diseases which needs constant care, mobility problems from old age or balance issues/orthopedic problems/CVAs, dementia, etc can all necessitate subacute rehabilitation or nursing home placement (w/ social workers help).

  1. Get PT/OT evaluation: to known where is the placement in: acute/subacute rehap or nursing home depends on their level of independability.

  2. Get PPD (must of nursing homes requires it)

  3. Ask the pt (or his/her family) about placement: as they need to agree on the placement plan. If they want to get the pt home no matter what, no need to start the process.

  4. Check the pt's insurance if it will cover the expenses

  5. Check the need for long-term IV meds like abx, what kind, O_2 need & feeding tube need, as they are all should be included in the application.

  6. Assure the need for transportation at the time of pt's discharge & check w/ the social worker if the hospital can arrange for one so you don't unnecessarily keep the pt for extra days in the hospital for just transportation.

Abbreviations

Term	Abbr.
Increase	↑
decrease	↓
Acute kidney injury	AKI
Alcohol	EtOH
and	&
Arterial blood gas	ABG
Atrial fibrillation	A fib
Biopsy	bx
Bone marrow	BM
Capillary blood glucose	CBG
Cardiovascular	CV
Chest pain	CP
Chest x-ray	CXR
Congestive heart failure	CHF
Coronary artery bypass surgery	CABG
Coronary artery disease	CAD
Culture	Cx
Diabetes mellitus	DM
diabetic ketoacidosis	DKA
Differential diagnosis	DDx
Dysfunction	Dysfx
Ejection fraction	EF
Electrocardiogram	EKG
End stage renal disease	ESRD

Term	Abbr.
Esophagus gastric duodenum	EGD
Headache	HA
Hemoglobin	Hgb
History	hx
Hyperosmolar hyperglycemic nonketotic syndrome	HHNS
Hypertension	HTN
Hypotension	HoTN
Herpes Zoster Virus	HZV
Infection	Infx
Intravenous	IV
Magnesium	Mg
Medical	MICU
Medication	meds
Myocardial infarction	MI
Nausea & vomiting	N/V
Nitroglycerin	NTG
Non ST elevation myocardial Infarction	NSTE MI
Oral	PO
patient	pt
Pneumonia	PNA
Pulmonary	Pulm
Reticulocyte index	RI
Serum creatinine	Cr

ST elevation myocardial Infarction	STEMI
Symptoms Sx	Sx
Treatment Tx	Tx
Urinary tract infection	UTI
Urine analysis	UA
Urine drug screen	UDS
Vacomycin	Vanc
With	w/
With out	w/o
beta blocker	B blocker
Mean artery pressure	MAP
Cardiac output	CO
Total peripheral resistance	TPR
Heart rate	HR
Stroke volume	SV
As needed	PRN
Left bundle branch block	LBBB
Right bundle branch block	RBBB
Aspirin	ASA
Gastroenterology	GI
CT angiography	CTA
Arterial blood gas	ABG
Deep venous thrombosis	DVT
Tissue Plasminogen	tPA
Jogular venous	JVD

distension	
Right ventricle	RV
Brain natriuretic peptide	BNP
Basic metabolic panel	BMP
Rapid plasma reagin	RPR
Infective endocarditis	IE
Anti nuclear antibodies	ANA
Anti-neutrophil cytoplasmic antibody	ANCA
Fecal occult blood test	FOBT
peripherally inserted central catheter	PICC line
Small bowel obstruction	SBO
Community acquired pneumonia	CAP
Healthcare acquired pneumonia	HCAP
Ventricular fibrillation	VF
Gram positive/negative	G+/-
Proton pumb inhipitor	PPI
Over the counter	OTC
Atriovenous malformation	AVM
Central nervous system	CNS
Cerebral vascular disease	CVA
Levt ventricular assist device	LVAT
Left anterior descending	LAD

128

Right coronary artery	RCA
Creatine phosphokinase	CPK
Patent foramen ovale	PFO
Drug-eluting stent	DES
partial pressure arterial oxygen	PaO2
fraction of inspired oxygen	FiO2
Acute respiratory distress syndrome	ARDS
glomerular basement membrane	GBM
Primary care provider	PCP
Benign prostatic hyperplasia	BPH
Non-invasive positive pressure ventilation	NIPPV or NIV
Fresh frozen plasma	FFP

Hydrochlorothiazide	HCTZ
Calcium channel blocker	CCB
Drug adverse effect	DAE
Pulmonary function test	PFT
Hemodialysis	HD
Hemoglobin	Hgb
Ventilation/perfusion	V/Q
Esophagogastroduodenoscopy	EGD
Transthoracic Echocardiogram	TTE
Dyspnia on exertion	DOE
Percutaneous coronary angiogram/intervention	PCA/PCI
Obstructive sleep apenia	OSA
Rule out	r/o
Anticoagulation	Antico-agx

List of medications commonly used

Brand	(Generic) Indication
Abilify	(Aripiprazole) Antipsychotic
Actonel	(Risedronate) Osteoporosis agent
Actos	(Pioglitazone) Antidiabetic
Advair	(Fluticasone + Salmeterol) Antiasthmatic
Aldactone	(Spirinolactone) <K+ sparing diuretic>
Allegra-D	(Fexofenadine + Pseudoephedrine) Antihistamine/ Decongestant
Ambien	(Zolpidem) Hypnotic sedative
Amoxil	(Amoxicillin) Penicillin Antibiotic
Flexeril	(Cyclobenzaprine) Muscle relaxant
Aleve	(Naproxen) NSAID
Antivert	(Meclizine) Anti-vertigo agent
Aricept	(Donepezil) Antipsychotic/ Agent for Alzheimer's Dementia
Atarax	(Hydroxyzine) Antianxiety/ Antipruritic
Ativan	(Lorazepam) Antianxiety
Augmentin	(Amoxicillin/ Clavulanate) Penicillin antibiotic w/ penicillinase inhibitor
Avandia	(Rosiglitazone) Antidiabetic
Avelox	(Moxifloxacin) Fluoroquinolone antibiotic
Avodart	(Dutasteride) Prostate anti-inflammatory
Bactrim, Septra	(Sulfamethoxazole/Trimethoprim) Sulfonamide antibiotic
Bactroban	(Mupirocin) Antibacterial <topical ointment>
Benadryl	(Diphenhydramine) Antihistamine
Benicar	(Olmesartan) Antihypertensive
Bentyl	(Dicyclomine) GI antispasmotic
Boniva	(Ibandronate) Osteoporosis agent

BuSpar	(Buspirone) Antianxiety agent
Capzasin-HP	(Capsaicin cream) Arthritis pain relief
Cardizem	(Diltiazem) Antihypertensive/anginal <non-DHP CCB>
Cardura	(Doxazosin) Antihypertensive/ BPH Agent <alpha-1 antagonist>
Catapres	(Clonidine) Antihypertensive <central α2-agonist>
Ceftin	(Cefuroxime) Cephalosporin Antibiotic 2nd G
Celebrex	(Celecoxib) NSAID, selective for COX2
Celexa	(Citalopram) Antidepressant SSRI
Chantix	(Varenicline) Smoking Cessation Aid
Cialis	(Tadalafil) Erectile dysftn
Cipro	(Ciprofloxacin) Fluoroquinolone antibiotic
Cleocin	(Clindamycin) Antibiotic
Cogentin	(Benztropine Mesylate) Anti-Parkinson
Colchicine	(generic only) anti-inflammotary for gout
Combivent	(Ipratropium + Albuterol MDI) Antiasthmatic
Cordarone	(Amiodarone) Antiarrhythmic <class III>
Coreg	(Carvedilol) Antihypertensive <nonselective beta-blocker with alpha-1 blocker)
Coumadin	(Warfarin) Anticoagulant
Cozaar	(Losartan) Antihypertensive
Crestor	(Rosuvastatin) Antihyperlipidemic, high potency <HMG-CoA reductase inhibitor>
Cymbalta	(Duloxetine) Antidepressant SNRI
Deltasone	(Prednisone) Anti-inflammatory
Depakote	(Divalproex) Antiepileptic/Antipsychotic

Desyrel	(Trazadone) Antidepressant
Detrol	(Tolterodine) Urinary bladder modifier
Diflucan	(Fluconazole) Antifungal
Dilantin Kapseals	(Phenytoin) Antiepileptic
Dilaudid	(Hydromorphone) Analgesic
Diovan	(Valsartan) Antihypertensive
Ditropan	(Oxybutynin) Urinary bladder modifier
Drisdol	(Vitamin D, Ergocalciferol) Vitamin
DuoNeb	(Ipratropium + Albuterol soln) Antiasthmatic
Duragesic	(Fentanyl) Opioid Analgesic
Dyazide, Maxzide	(Triamtrene/ HCTZ) Diuretic <K+ sparing + thiazide diuretic>
Ecotrin	(Aspirin, enteric-coated) Blood Modifier <platelet inhibitor>
Effexor	(Venlafaxine) Antidepressant SNRI
Effient	(Prasurgel) antiplatelets, used similar to plavix.
Elavil	(Amitriptyline) Antidepressant TCA
Eliquis	(ApiXaban) inhibit Factor X, novel oral anticoagx
Estrace	(Estradiol) Estrogen hormone, gel/tab/patch/vaginal/IM
Evista	(Raloxifene) Osteoporosis agent
Flagyl	(Metronidazole) Antibacterial/ Antiprotozoal
Flomax	(Tamsulosin) for BPH <alpha 1-a selective blocker>
Flonase	(Fluticasone) Antiallergy
Flovent	(Fluticasone MDI) Antiasthmatic
Fosamax	(Alendronate) Osteoporosis agent
Glucophage	(Metformin) Antidiabetic
Glucotrol	(Glipizide) Antidiabetic

Glucovance	(Glyburide/ Metformin) Antidiabetic
Haldol	(Haloperidol) Antipsychotic
Humalog	(Insulin Lispro, rDNA origin) Anti-diabetic
Humulin N, Humulin R	(Regular insulin NPH, Regular insulin) Anti-diabetic
HydroDiuril	(Hydrochlorothiazide) Thiazide Diuretic
Hytrin	(Terazosin) Antihypertensive/BPH <beta-1 antagonist>
Hyzaar	(Losartan + HCT) Antihypertensive
Imdur	(Isosorbide mononitrate) Antianginal
Integrilin	(Eptifibatide), anti-platelets, used mainly in PCI. Blocks binding of fibrinogen & von Willebrand factor to glycoprotein IIb/IIIa receptor on platelet surface
Isordil	(Isosorbide dinonitrate) Antianginal
Isoptin	(Verapimil) Antihypertensive/ Antianginal
Januvia	(Sitagliptin) Antidiabetic
Keflex	(Cephalexin) Cephalosporin antibiotic
Kenalog	(Tiramcinolone Acetonide) Topical Corticosteroid
Keppra	(Levetiracetam) Anti-convulsant
Klonopin	(Clonazepam) Antiepileptic
Lamicatal	(Lamotrigine) Antiepileptic
Lanoxin	(Digoxin) Inotropic agent
Lantus	(Insulin Glargine) Anti-diabetic
Lasix	(Furosemide) Loop Diuretic
Levaquin	(Levofloxacin) Fluoroquinolone antibiotic
Lexapro	(Escitalopram) Antidepressant SSRI
Lioresal	(Baclofen) Muscle relaxant
Lipitor	(Atorvastatin) Antihyperlipidemic, high potency <HMG-CoA reductase

inhibitor>

Lopid	(Gemfibrozil) Antihyperlipidemic <activate PPARa>
Lopressor	(Metoprolol Tartrate) Antihypertensive < B blocker>
Lortab, Vicodin	(Hydrocodone w/ tylenol) Opioid Analgesic
Lotensin	(Benazepril) Antihypertensive <ACE Inhibitor>
Lotrisone	(Clotrimazole w/ Betamethasone) Topical Antifungal
Lovaza	(Omega-3 FAs) Antihyperlipidemic
Lyrica	(Pregabalin) Anti-convulsant/Antineuralgic
Macrodantin, Macrobid	(Nitrofurantoin) Antibacterial
Medrol	(Methylpredisolone) Anti-inflammatory
Methadose, Dolophine	(Methadone) Opioid Analgesic
Micronase	(Glyburide) Antidiabetic
Miralax	(Polyethylene Glycol 2250) Laxative
Mobic	(Meloxicam) NSAID, non-selective COX inhipitor
Motrin	(Ibuprofen) NSAID
MS Contin	(Morphine Sulfate) Opioid Analgesic, long acting
Mytussin AC, Robutussin AC	(Codeine Phosphate w/ Guaifenesin) Antitussive/Expectorant
Namenda	(Memantine) Agent for Alzheimer's Dementia
Nasacort AQ	(Triamcinolone) Antiallergy
Nasonex	(Mometasone) Antiallergy
Neurontin	(Gabapentin) Antiepileptic, for neuropathy as well.
Nexium	(Esomeprazole) PPI

Niaspan	(Niacin) Antihyperlipidemic <increase lipoprotein lipase activity>
Nitrostat	(Nitroglycerin) Antianginal
Nizoral	(Ketoconazole) Antifungal
Norvasc	(Amlopidine) Antihypertensive <DHP CCB>
Novolog	(Insulin Aspart, rDNA origin) Anti-diabetic
NuvaRing	(Etonogestrel & Ethinyl estradiol) Contraceptive
Nystop	(Nystatin) Antifungal Antibiotic
Omnicef	(Cefdinir) Cephalosporin antibiotic, PO 3rd G
Oraped	(Prednisolone) Anti-inflammatory
Othro-Cyclen, Sprintec	(Norgestimate & Ethinyl estradiol) Oral contraceptive
Ovral, Lo/Ovral, Ogestrel,	(Noregestrel & Ethinyl estradiol) Oral contraceptive
Oxycontin	(Oxycodone CR) Opioid Analgesic
OxyIR, Roxicodone	(Oxycodone IR) Opioid Analgesic
Pamelor	(Nortriptyline) Antidepressant TCA
Paxil	(Paroxetine) Antidepressant SSRI
Pepcid	(Famotadine) Anti-ulcer agent
Percocet	(Oxycodone w/ tylenol) Opioid Analgesic
Phenergan	(Promethazine) Anti-emetic
Plaquenil	(Hydroxychloroquine) Antimalarial
Plavix	(Clopidogrel) Platelet Inhibitor
Pradaxa	(Dabigatran) inhibit thrombin, novel anticoagx
Pravachol	(Pravastatin) Antihyperlipidemic <HMG-CoA reductase inhibitor>
Premarin	(Conjugated estrogens) Estrogen

	Hormone
Prilosec	(Omeprazole) Anti-ulcer agent
Procardia, Nifedical, Adalet	(Nifedipine) Antihypertensive/ Antianginal <DHP CCB>
Proscar	(Finasteride) Prostate anti-inflammatory
Protonix	(Pantoprazole) Anti-ulcer agent
Proventil, Ventolin, Proair	(Albuterol) Anti-asthmatic
Prozac	(Fluoxetine) Antidepressant SSRI
Pyridium	(Phenazopyridine) Urinary tract analgesic
Ranexa	(Ranolazine) 2nd line anti-anginal, unknown mechanism.
Reglan	(Metoclopramide) Anti-emetic
Remeron	(Mirtazapine) Antidepressant
Requip	(Ropinirole) Anti-Parkinson, restless leg syndrome
Risperdal	(Risperidone) Antipsychotic
Robaxin	(Methocarbamol) Muscle relaxant
Seroquel	(Quetiapine) Antipsychotic
Singulair	(Montelukast) Antiasthmatic
Soma	(Carisoprodol) Muscle relaxant
Spiriva	(Tiotropium) Antiasthmatic
Suboxone	(Buprenorphine w/ Naloxone) Agent for Opioid Dependence
Synthroid, Levothyroid	(Levothyroxine) Thyroid hormone
Tamiflu	(Oseltamivir) Antiviral
Temovate	(Clobetasol Proprionate) Topical Anti-inflammatory
Tessalon	(Benzonatate) Antitussive
Topamax	(Topiramate) Antiepileptic

Toprol-XL	(Metoprolol Succinate) Antihypertensive <selective beta-1 blocker>
Tricor	(Fenofibrate) Antihyperlipidemic (mainly TG)
Tussionex	(Clorpheniramine w/ Hydrocodone) Antitussive
Ultram, Ryzolt	(Tramadol HCl) Analgesic
Valium	(Diazepam) Antianxiety
Valtrex	(Valacyclovir) Antiviral
Veramyst	(Fluticasone) Antiallergy
Viagra	(Sildenafil) Erectile dysftn
Victosa	(Liraglutide) SQ meds for DMII & obesity, increase insulin
Vibramycin	(Doxycycline) Tetracycline antibiotic
Avelox	(Moxifloxacin) Fluoroquinolone antibiotic
Vivelle-Dot	(Estradiol) Hormonal replacement <topical>
Voltaren	(Diclofenac) NSAID
Wellbutrin	(Bupropion) Antidepressant
Xanax	(Alprazolam) Antianxiety
Xarelto	(RivaroXaban) inhibit Factor X, novel oral anticoagx.
Xopenex	(Levalbuterol) Antiasthmatic
Yasmin, Ocella	(Drospirenone & Ethinyl estradiol) Oral contraceptive
Zanaflex	(Tizanidine) Muscle relaxant
Zantac	(Ranitidine) Anti-ulcer agent
Zebeta	(Bisoprolol) Antihypertensive
Zestril	(Lisinopril) Antihypertensive <ACE Inhibitor>
Zetia	(Ezetimibe) Antihyperlipidemic <inhibits intestinal absorption of cholesterol>

Zithromax, Z pack	(Azithromycin) Macrolide Antibiotic
Zocor	(Simvastatin) Antihyperlipidemic <HMG-CoA reductase inhibitor>
Zoloft	(Sertraline) Antidepressant SSRI
Zosyn	(Piperacillin/tazobactam) Antibiotic
Zovirax	(Acyclovir) Antiviral
Zyloprim	(Allopurinol) Agent for gout
Zyprexa	(Olanzapine) Atypical Antipsychotic

References

1.	Harrison's Principles of Internal Medicine, 18th edition. Dan L. Longo, Editor, Anthony S. Fauci, Editor, Dennis L. Kasper, Editor, Stephen L. Hauser, Editor, J. Larry Jameson, Editor, Joseph Loscalzo, Editor

2.	Foster C, Misry NF, Peddi PF, Sharma S. The Washington Manual of Medical Therapeutics. 33rd edition. Department of Medicine, Washington University School of Medicine. Wolters Kluwer/Lippincott Williams & Wilkins; 2010.

3.	Sabatine MS. Pocket Medicine (The Massachusetts General Hospital Handbook of Internal Medicine). Fourth Edition. Wolters Kluwer/Lippincott Williams & Wilkins; 2010.

4.	Pavlik VN, Hyman DJ, Wendt JA, Orengo C. Association of a culturally defined syndrome (nervios) with chest pain and DSM-IV affective disorders in Hispanic patients referred for cardiac stress testing. Ethn Dis 2004; 14:505.

5.	Challenging existing paradigms in ischemic heart disease: the NHBLI-sponsored women's ischemia syndrome evaluation (WISE). J Am Coll Cardiol 2006; 47:1S.

6.	D'Antono B, Dupuis G, Fortin C, et al. Angina symptoms in men and women with stable coronary artery disease and evidence of exercise-induced myocardial perfusion defects. Am Heart J 2006; 151:813.

7.	von Kodolitsch Y, Schwartz AG, Nienaber CA. Clinical prediction of acute aortic dissection. Arch Intern Med 2000; 160:2977.

8.	McGee, S. Pulmonary embolism. In: Evidence based physical diagnosis, 2, Saunders Elsevier, 2007. p.365.

9.	Marcus GM, Cohen J, Varosy PD, et al. The utility of gestures in patients with chest discomfort. Am J Med 2007; 120:83.

10.	Davies HA, Jones DB, Rhodes J, Newcombe RG. Angina-like esophageal pain: differentiation from cardiac pain by history. J Clin Gastroenterol 1985; 7:477. DWORKEN HJ, BIEL FJ, MACHELLA TE. Supradiaphragmatic reference of pain from the colon. Gastroenterology 1952; 22:222.

11.	Ryle JA. Visceral pain and referred pain. Lancet 1926; 1:895.

12.	Selzer M, Spencer WA. Convergence of visceral and cutaneous afferent pathways in the lumbar spinal cord. Brain Res 1969; 14:331.

13.	Purcell TB. Nonsurgical and extraperitoneal causes of abdominal pain. Emerg Med Clin North Am 1989; 7:721.

14.	Saik RP, Greenburg AG, Farris JM, Peskin GW. Spectrum of cholangitis. Am J Surg 1975; 130:143.

15.	Go VL, Everhart JE. Pancreatitis. In: Digestive diseases in the United States: Epidemiology and impact, Everhart JE (Ed), National Institutes of Health, National Institute of Diabetes and Digestive and Kidney Diseases. US Government Printing Office, Washington, DC 1994. p.693.

16.	Talley NJ, Colin-Jones D, Koch KL, et al. Functional dyspepsia: A classification with guidelines for diagnosis and management. Gastroenterol Int 1992; 4:145.

17.	Flanagin BA, Mitchell MT, Thistlethwaite WA, Alverdy JC. Diagnosis and treatment of atypical presentations of hiatal hernia following bariatric surgery. Obes Surg 2010; 20:386.

18.	Beeson MS. Splenic infarct presenting as acute abdominal pain in an older patient. J Emerg Med 1996; 14:319.

19.	Nores M, Phillips EH, Morgenstern L, Hiatt JR. The clinical spectrum of splenic infarction. Am Surg 1998; 64:182.

20.	Franklin QJ, Compeggie M. Splenic syndrome in sickle cell trait: four case presentations and a review of the literature. Mil Med 1999; 164:230.

21.	Görg C, Seifart U, Görg K. Acute, complete splenic infarction in cancer patient is associated with a fatal outcome. Abdom Imaging 2004; 29:224. Hung JJ, Hsu HS, Huang CS, Yang KY. Tracheoesophageal fistula and tracheo-subclavian artery fistula after tracheostomy. Eur J Cardiothorac Surg 2007; 32:676.

22.	Komatsu T, Sowa T, Fujinaga T, et al. Tracheo-innominate artery fistula: two case reports and a clinical review. Ann Thorac Cardiovasc Surg 2013; 19:60.

23.	Choudhary C, Bandyopadhyay D, Salman R, et al. Broncho-vascular fistulas from self-expanding metallic stents: A retrospective case review. Ann Thorac Med 2013; 8:116.

24.	Savale L, Parrot A, Khalil A, et al. Cryptogenic hemoptysis: from a benign to a life-threatening pathologic vascular condition. Am J Respir Crit Care Med 2007; 175:1181.

25.	Kuzucu A, Gürses I, Soysal O, et al. Dieulafoy's disease: a cause of massive hemoptysis that is probably underdiagnosed. Ann Thorac Surg 2005; 80:1126.

26.	Kolb T, Gilbert C, Fishman EK, et al. Dieulafoy's disease of the bronchus. Am J Respir Crit Care Med 2012; 186:1191.

27.	Muniappan A, Tapias LF, Butala P, et al. Surgical therapy of pulmonary aspergillomas: a 30-year North American experience. Ann Thorac Surg 2014; 97:432.

28.	Farid S, Mohamed S, Devbhandari M, et al. Results of surgery for chronic pulmonary Aspergillosis, optimal antifungal therapy and proposed high risk factors for recurrence--a National Centre's experience. J Cardiothorac Surg 2013; 8:180.

29.	Ahmed S, Mohammad VW, Hamid F, et al. The 2011 dengue haemorrhagic fever outbreak in Lahore - an account of clinical parameters and pattern of haemorrhagic complications. J Coll Physicians Surg Pak 2013; 23:463.

30.	Sareli AE, Janssen WJ, Sterman D, et al. Clinical problem-solving. What's the connection? - A 26-year-old white man presented to our referral hospital with a 1-month history of persistent cough productive of white sputum, which was occasionally tinged with blood. N Engl J Med 2008; 358:626.

31.	Drent M, Wessels S, Jacobs JA, Thijssen H. Association of diffuse alveolar haemorrhage with acquired vitamin K deficiency. Respiration 2000; 67:697.

32.	Ikeda M, Tanaka H, Sadamatsu K. Diffuse alveolar hemorrhage as a complication of dual antiplatelet therapy for acute coronary syndrome. Cardiovasc Revasc Med 2011; 12:407.

33.	Chen BC, Sheth NR, Dadzie KA, et al. Hemodialysis for the treatment of pulmonary hemorrhage from dabigatran overdose. Am J Kidney Dis 2013; 62:591.

34.	Heck SL, Blom P, Berstad A. Accuracy and complications in computed tomography fluoroscopy-guided needle biopsies of lung masses. Eur Radiol 2006; 16:1387.
35.	Choi JW, Park CM, Goo JM, et al. C-arm cone-beam CT-guided percutaneous transthoracic needle biopsy of small (≤ 20 mm) lung nodules: diagnostic accuracy and complications in 161 patients. AJR Am J Roentgenol 2012; 199:W322.
36.	Lee SM, Park CM, Lee KH, et al. C-arm cone-beam CT-guided percutaneous transthoracic needle biopsy of lung nodules: clinical experience in 1108 patients. Radiology 2014; 271:291.
37.	Augoulea A, Lambrinoudaki I, Christodoulakos G. Thoracic endometriosis syndrome. Respiration 2008; 75:113.
38.	Sandler A, Gray R, Perry MC, et al. Paclitaxel-carboplatin alone or with bevacizumab for non-small-cell lung cancer. N Engl J Med 2006; 355:2542.
39.	Cho YJ, Murgu SD, Colt HG. Bronchoscopy for bevacizumab-related hemoptysis. Lung Cancer 2007; 56:465.
40.	Karlson-Stiber C, Höjer J, Sjöholm A, et al. Nitrogen dioxide pneumonitis in ice hockey players. J Intern Med 1996; 239:451.
41.	Centers for Disease Control and Prevention (CDC). Exposure to nitrogen dioxide in an indoor ice arena - New Hampshire, 2011. MMWR Morb Mortal Wkly Rep 2012; 61:139. American College of Cardiology Foundation, American Heart Association, European Society of Cardiology, et al. Management of patients with atrial fibrillation (compilation of 2006 ACCF/AHA/ESC and 2011 ACCF/AHA/HRS recommendations): a report of the American College of Cardiology/American Heart Association Task Force on practice guidelines. Circulation 2013; 127:1916.
42.	January CT, Wann LS, Alpert JS, et al. 2014 AHA/ACC/HRS guideline for the management of patients with atrial fibrillation: a report of the American College of Cardiology/American Heart Association Task Force on practice guidelines and the Heart Rhythm Society. Circulation 2014; 130:e199.
43.	January CT, Wann LS, Alpert JS, et al. 2014 AHA/ACC/HRS guideline for the management of patients with atrial fibrillation: executive summary: a report of the American College of Cardiology/American Heart Association Task Force on practice guidelines and the Heart Rhythm Society. Circulation 2014; 130:2071.
44.	Wyse DG, Van Gelder IC, Ellinor PT, et al. Lone atrial fibrillation: does it exist? J Am Coll Cardiol 2014; 63:1715.
45.	Kopecky SL, Gersh BJ, McGoon MD, et al. The natural history of lone atrial fibrillation. A population-based study over three decades. N Engl J Med 1987; 317:669.
46.	Brand FN, Abbott RD, Kannel WB, Wolf PA. Characteristics and prognosis of lone atrial fibrillation. 30-year follow-up in the Framingham Study. JAMA 1985; 254:3449.
47.	Kannel WB, Abbott RD, Savage DD, McNamara PM. Epidemiologic features of chronic atrial fibrillation: the Framingham study. N Engl J Med 1982; 306:1018.
48.	Lévy S, Maarek M, Coumel P, et al. Characterization of different subsets of atrial fibrillation in general practice in France: the ALFA study. The College of French Cardiologists. Circulation 1999; 99:3028.
49.	Takahashi N, Seki A, Imataka K, Fujii J. Clinical features of paroxysmal atrial fibrillation. An observation of 94 patients. Jpn Heart J 1981; 22:143.
50.	Clementy J, Dulhoste MN, Laiter C, et al. Flecainide acetate in the prevention of paroxysmal atrial fibrillation: a nine-month follow-up of more than 500 patients. Am J Cardiol 1992; 70:44A.
51.	EVANS W, SWANN P. Lone auricular fibrillation. Br Heart J 1954; 16:189.
52.	LAMB LE, POLLARD LW. ATRIAL FIBRILLATION IN FLYING PERSONNEL. Circulation 1964; 29:694.
53.	Peter RH, Gracey JG, Beach TB. A clinical profile of idiopathic atrial fibrillation. A functional disorder of atrial rhythm. Ann Intern Med 1968; 68:1288.
54.	Rostagno C, Bacci F, Martelli M, et al. Clinical course of lone atrial fibrillation since first symptomatic arrhythmic episode. Am J Cardiol 1995; 76:837. Sterns RH, Silver SM. Salt and water: read the package insert. QJM 2003; 96:549.
55.	Rose BD, Post TW. Clinical Physiology of Acid-Base and Electrolyte Disorders, 5th ed, McGraw-Hill, New York 2001. p.441.
56.	Lu KC, Hsu YJ, Chiu JS, et al. Effects of potassium supplementation on the recovery of thyrotoxic periodic paralysis. Am J Emerg Med 2004; 22:544.
57.	McCowen KC, Malhotra A, Bistrian BR. Stress-induced hyperglycemia. Crit Care Clin 2001; 17:107. tension. J Appl Physiol Respir Environ Exerc Physiol 1981; 57:686.
58.	Taguchi O, Kikuchi Y, Hida W, et al. Effects of bronchoconstriction and external resistive loading on the sensation of dyspnea. J Appl Physiol (1985) 1991; 71:2183.
59.	Moy ML, Woodrow Weiss J, Sparrow D, et al. Quality of dyspnea in bronchoconstriction differs from external resistive loads. Am J Respir Crit Care Med 2000; 162:451.
60.	Clark AL, Piepoli M, Coats AJ. Skeletal muscle and the control of ventilation on exercise: evidence for metabolic receptors. Eur J Clin Invest 1995; 25:299.
61.	Clark A, Volterrani M, Swan JW, et al. Leg blood flow, metabolism and exercise capacity in chronic stable heart failure. Int J Cardiol 1996; 55:127.
62.	Killian KJ, Leblanc P, Martin DH, et al. Exercise capacity and ventilatory, circulatory, and symptom limitation in patients with chronic airflow limitation. Am Rev Respir Dis 1992; 146:935.
63.	Melzack R, Torgerson WS. On the language of pain. Anesthesiology 1971; 34:50.
64.	Melzack R. The McGill Pain Questionnaire: major properties and scoring methods. Pain 1975; 1:277.
65.	Hunter M, Philips C. The experience of headache pain--an assessment of the qualities of tension headache pain. Pain 1981; 10:209. Netea MG, Kullberg BJ, Van der Meer JW. Circulating cytokines as mediators of fever. Clin Infect Dis 2000; 31 Suppl 5:S178.
66.	Blatteis CM, Sehic E, Li S. Pyrogen sensing and signaling: old views and new concepts. Clin Infect Dis 2000; 31 Suppl 5:S168.
67.	Saper CB, Breder CD. The neurologic basis of fever. N Engl J Med 1994; 330:1880.
68.	Mitchell, JD, Grocott, HP, Phillips-Bute, B, et al. Cytokine secretion after cardiac surgery and its relationship to postoperative fever. Cytokine 2007; 39:37.
69.	Dauleh MI, Rahman S, Townell NH. Open versus laparoscopic cholecystectomy: a comparison of postoperative temperature. J R Coll Surg Edinb 1995; 40:116.

70.   Clark JA, Bar-Yosef S, Anderson A, et al. Postoperative hyperthermia following off-pump versus on-pump coronary artery bypass surgery. J Cardiothorac Vasc Anesth 2005; 19:426.
71.   Ghert M, Allen B, Davids J, et al. Increased postoperative febrile response in children with osteogenesis imperfecta. J Pediatr Orthop 2003; 23:261. Rocha-Singh KJ, Eisenhauer AC, Textor SC, et al. Atherosclerotic Peripheral Vascular Disease Symposium II: intervention for renal artery disease. Circulation 2008; 118:2873.
72.   Bortman G, Sellanes M, Odell DS, et al. Discrepancy between pre- and post-transplant diagnosis of end-stage dilated cardiomyopathy. Am J Cardiol 1994; 74:921.
73.   Marwick TH. The viable myocardium: epidemiology, detection, and clinical implications. Lancet 1998; 351:815.
74.   Allman KC, Shaw LJ, Hachamovitch R, Udelson JE. Myocardial viability testing and impact of revascularization on prognosis in patients with coronary artery disease and left ventricular dysfunction: a meta-analysis. J Am Coll Cardiol 2002; 39:1151.
75.   Repetto A, Dal Bello B, Pasotti M, et al. Coronary atherosclerosis in end-stage idiopathic dilated cardiomyopathy: an innocent bystander? Eur Heart J 2005; 26:1519.
76.   Jessup M, Brozena S. Heart failure. N Engl J Med 2003; 348:2007.
77.   Koelling TM, Aaronson KD, Cody RJ, et al. Prognostic significance of mitral regurgitation and tricuspid regurgitation in patients with left ventricular systolic dysfunction. Am Heart J 2002; 144:524.
78.   Fonarow GC, Yancy CW, Hernandez AF, et al. Potential impact of optimal implementation of evidence-based heart failure therapies on mortality. Am Heart J 2011; 161:1024.
79.   Willenheimer R, van Veldhuisen DJ, Silke B, et al. Effect on survival and hospitalization of initiating treatment for chronic heart failure with bisoprolol followed by enalapril, as compared with the opposite sequence: results of the randomized Cardiac Insufficiency Bisoprolol Study (CIBIS) III. Circulation 2005; 112:2426.
80.   Sliwa K, Norton GR, Kone N, et al. Impact of initiating carvedilol before angiotensin-converting enzyme inhibitor therapy on cardiac function in newly diagnosed heart failure. J Am Coll Cardiol 2004; 44:1825.
81.   Fang JC. Angiotensin-converting enzyme inhibitors or beta-blockers in heart failure: does it matter who goes first? Circulation 2005; 112:2380.
82.   Bristow MR, Gilbert EM, Abraham WT, et al. Carvedilol produces dose-related improvements in left ventricular function and survival in subjects with chronic heart failure. MOCHA Investigators. Circulation 1996; 94:2807.
83.   Wikstrand J, Hjalmarson A, Waagstein F, et al. Dose of metoprolol CR/XL and clinical outcomes in patients with heart failure: analysis of the experience in metoprolol CR/XL randomized intervention trial in chronic heart failure (MERIT-HF). J Am Coll Cardiol 2002; 40:491.
84.   Faris R, Flather MD, Purcell H, et al. Diuretics for heart failure. Cochrane Database Syst Rev 2006; :CD003838.
85.   Effect of enalapril on mortality and the development of heart failure in asymptomatic patients with reduced left ventricular ejection fractions. The SOLVD Investigattors. N Engl J Med 1992; 327:685.
86.   Cohn JN, Johnson G, Ziesche S, et al. A comparison of enalapril with hydralazine-isosorbide dinitrate in the treatment of chronic congestive heart failure. N Engl J Med 1991; 325:303.
87.   Effects of enalapril on mortality in severe congestive heart failure. Results of the Cooperative North Scandinavian Enalapril Survival Study (CONSENSUS). The CONSENSUS Trial Study Group. N Engl J Med 1987; 316:1429.
88.   Effect of enalapril on survival in patients with reduced left ventricular ejection fractions and congestive heart failure. The SOLVD Investigators. N Engl J Med 1991; 325:293.
89.   Flather MD, Yusuf S, Køber L, et al. Long-term ACE-inhibitor therapy in patients with heart failure or left-ventricular dysfunction: a systematic overview of data from individual patients. ACE-Inhibitor Myocardial Infarction Collaborative Group. Lancet 2000; 355:1575.
90.   Kostis JB, Shelton BJ, Yusuf S, et al. Tolerability of enalapril initiation by patients with left ventricular dysfunction: results of the medication challenge phase of the Studies of Left Ventricular Dysfunction. Am Heart J 1994; 128:358.
91.   Packer M, Poole-Wilson PA, Armstrong PW, et al. Comparative effects of low and high doses of the angiotensin-converting enzyme inhibitor, lisinopril, on morbidity and mortality in chronic heart failure. ATLAS Study Group. Circulation 1999; 100:2312.
92.   Delahaye F, de Gevigney G. Is the optimal dose of angiotensin-converting enzyme inhibitors in patients with congestive heart failure definitely established? J Am Coll Cardiol 2000; 36:2096.
93.   Brophy JM, Joseph L, Rouleau JL. Beta-blockers in congestive heart failure. A Bayesian meta-analysis. Ann Intern Med 2001; 134:550.
94.   Effect of metoprolol CR/XL in chronic heart failure: Metoprolol CR/XL Randomised Intervention Trial in Congestive Heart Failure (MERIT-HF). Lancet 1999; 353:2001. Ahmed A, Rich MW, Fleg JL, et al. Effects of digoxin on morbidity and mortality in diastolic heart failure: the ancillary digitalis investigation group trial. Circulation 2006; 114:397.
95.   Digitalis Investigation Group. The effect of digoxin on mortality and morbidity in patients with heart failure. N Engl J Med 1997; 336:525.
96.   ALLHAT Officers and Coordinators for the ALLHAT Collaborative Research Group. The Antihypertensive and Lipid-Lowering Treatment to Prevent Heart Attack Trial. Major outcomes in high-risk hypertensive patients randomized to angiotensin-converting enzyme inhibitor or calcium channel blocker vs diuretic: The Antihypertensive and Lipid-Lowering Treatment to Prevent Heart Attack Trial (ALLHAT). JAMA 2002; 288:2981.
97.   Beckett NS, Peters R, Fletcher AE, et al. Treatment of hypertension in patients 80 years of age or older. N Engl J Med 2008; 358:1887.
98.   Wachtell K, Bella JN, Rokkedal J, et al. Change in diastolic left ventricular filling after one year of antihypertensive treatment: The Losartan Intervention For Endpoint Reduction in Hypertension (LIFE) Study. Circulation 2002; 105:1071.
99.   Klingbeil AU, Schneider M, Martus P, et al. A meta-analysis of the effects of treatment on left ventricular mass in essential hypertension. Am J Med 2003; 115:41.
100. Bonow RO, Udelson JE. Left ventricular diastolic dysfunction as a cause of congestive heart failure. Mechanisms and management. Ann Intern Med 1992; 117:502.

141

101. Brutsaert DL, Sys SU, Gillebert TC. Diastolic failure: pathophysiology and therapeutic implications. J Am Coll Cardiol 1993; 22:318.
102. Bergström A, Andersson B, Edner M, et al. Effect of carvedilol on diastolic function in patients with diastolic heart failure and preserved systolic function. Results of the Swedish Doppler-echocardiographic study (SWEDIC). Eur J Heart Fail 2004; 6:453.
103. Andersson B, Caidahl K, di Lenarda A, et al. Changes in early and late diastolic filling patterns induced by long-term adrenergic beta-blockade in patients with idiopathic dilated cardiomyopathy. Circulation 1996; 94:673.
104. Poulsen SH, Jensen SE, Egstrup K. Effects of long-term adrenergic beta-blockade on left ventricular diastolic filling in patients with acute myocardial infarction. Am Heart J 1999; 138:710.
105. Flather MD, Shibata MC, Coats AJ, et al. Randomized trial to determine the effect of nebivolol on mortality and cardiovascular hospital admission in elderly patients with heart failure (SENIORS). Eur Heart J 2005; 26:215. Khalid S, Murdoch R, Newlands A, et al. Transient receptor potential vanilloid 1 (TRPV1) antagonism in patients with refractory chronic cough: a double-blind randomized controlled trial. J Allergy Clin Immunol 2014; 134:56.
106. Morice A, Kastelik JA, Thompson RH. Gender differences in airway behaviour. Thorax 2000; 55:629.
107. Kastelik JA, Thompson RH, Aziz I, et al. Sex-related differences in cough reflex sensitivity in patients with chronic cough. Am J Respir Crit Care Med 2002; 166:961.
108. Morice AH, Kastelik JA. Cough. 1: Chronic cough in adults. Thorax 2003; 58:901.
109. Kastelik JA, Aziz I, Ojoo JC, et al. Investigation and management of chronic cough using a probability-based algorithm. Eur Respir J 2005; 25:235.
110. Irwin RS, Madison JM. The diagnosis and treatment of cough. N Engl J Med 2000; 343:1715.
111. Pratter MR, Bartter T, Akers S, DuBois J. An algorithmic approach to chronic cough. Ann Intern Med 1993; 119:977.
112. Mello CJ, Irwin RS, Curley FJ. Predictive values of the character, timing, and complications of chronic cough in diagnosing its cause. Arch Intern Med 1996; 156:997.
113. McGarvey LP, Heaney LG, Lawson JT, et al. Evaluation and outcome of patients with chronic non-productive cough using a comprehensive diagnostic protocol. Thorax 1998; 53:738.
114. Iyer VN, Lim KG. Chronic cough: an update. Mayo Clin Proc 2013; 88:1115.
115. Kwon NH, Oh MJ, Min TH, et al. Causes and clinical features of subacute cough. Chest 2006; 129:1142.
116. Birring SS. Controversies in the evaluation and management of chronic cough. Am J Respir Crit Care Med 2011; 183:708.
117. Patrick H, Patrick F. Chronic cough. Med Clin North Am 1995; 79:361.
118. Pratter MR, Bartter T, Lotano R. The role of sinus imaging in the treatment of chronic cough in adults. Chest 1999; 116:1287.
119. Holinger LD, Sanders AD. Chronic cough in infants and children: an update. Laryngoscope 1991; 101:596.
120. Corrao WM, Braman SS, Irwin RS. Chronic cough as the sole presenting manifestation of bronchial asthma. N Engl J Med 1979; 300:633.
121. Johnson D, Osborn LM. Cough variant asthma: a review of the clinical literature. J Asthma 1991; 28:85.
122. O'Connell EJ, Rojas AR, Sachs MI. Cough-type asthma: a review. Ann Allergy 1991; 66:278.
123. Nakajima T, Nishimura Y, Nishiuma T, et al. Characteristics of patients with chronic cough who developed classic asthma during the course of cough variant asthma: a longitudinal study. Respiration 2005; 72:606.
124. McFadden ER Jr. Exertional dyspnea and cough as preludes to acute attacks of bronchial asthma. N Engl J Med 1975; 292:555.
125. Niimi A, Matsumoto H, Mishima M. Eosinophilic airway disorders associated with chronic cough. Pulm Pharmacol Ther 2009; 22:114.
126. Oh MJ, Lee JY, Lee BJ, Choi DC. Exhaled nitric oxide measurement is useful for the exclusion of nonasthmatic eosinophilic bronchitis in patients with chronic cough. Chest 2008; 134:990.
127. Hahn PY, Morgenthaler TY, Lim KG. Use of exhaled nitric oxide in predicting response to inhaled corticosteroids for chronic cough. Mayo Clin Proc 2007; 82:1350.
128. Prieto L, Ferrer A, Ponce S, et al. Exhaled nitric oxide measurement is NOT useful for predicting the response to inhaled corticosteroids in subjects with chronic cough. Chest 2009; 136:816.
129. Poe RH, Kallay MC. Chronic cough and gastroesophageal reflux disease: experience with specific therapy for diagnosis and treatment. Chest 2003; 123:679. White CW, Wright CB, Doty DB, et al. Does visual interpretation of the coronary arteriogram predict the physiologic importance of a coronary stenosis? N Engl J Med 1984; 310:819.
130. Ringqvist I, Fisher LD, Mock M, et al. Prognostic value of angiographic indices of coronary artery disease from the Coronary Artery Surgery Study (CASS). J Clin Invest 1983; 71:1854.
131. Emond M, Mock MB, Davis KB, et al. Long-term survival of medically treated patients in the Coronary Artery Surgery Study (CASS) Registry. Circulation 1994; 90:2645.
132. Gibbons RJ, Abrams J, Chatterjee K, et al. ACC/AHA 2002 guideline update for the management of patients with chronic stable angina www.acc.org/qualityandscience/clinical/statements.htm (Accessed on August 24, 2006).
133. Teo KK, Yusuf S, Furberg CD. Effects of prophylactic antiarrhythmic drug therapy in acute myocardial infarction. An overview of results from randomized controlled trials. JAMA 1993; 270:1589.
134. Braunwald E. Mechanism of action of calcium-channel-blocking agents. N Engl J Med 1982; 307:1618.
135. Heidenreich PA, McDonald KM, Hastie T, et al. Meta-analysis of trials comparing beta-blockers, calcium antagonists, and nitrates for stable angina. JAMA 1999; 281:1927.
136. Emanuelsson H, Egstrup K, Nikus K, et al. Antianginal efficacy of the combination of felodipine-metoprolol 10/100 mg compared with each drug alone in patients with stable effort-induced angina pectoris: a multicenter parallel group study. The TRAFFIC Study Group. Am Heart J 1999; 137:854.
137. Chaitman BR. Ranolazine for the treatment of chronic angina and potential use in other cardiovascular conditions. Circulation 2006; 113:2462.

138. Abrams J, Thadani U. Therapy of stable angina pectoris: the uncomplicated patient. Circulation 2005; 112:e255.
139. Winniford MD, Jansen DE, Reynolds GA, et al. Cigarette smoking-induced coronary vasoconstriction in atherosclerotic coronary artery disease and prevention by calcium antagonists and nitroglycerin. Am J Cardiol 1987; 59:203.
140. Winniford MD, Wheelan KR, Kremers MS, et al. Smoking-induced coronary vasoconstriction in patients with atherosclerotic coronary artery disease: evidence for adrenergically mediated alterations in coronary artery tone. Circulation 1986; 73:662.
141. van den Heuvel AF, Dunselman PH, Kingma T, et al. Reduction of exercise-induced myocardial ischemia during add-on treatment with the angiotensin-converting enzyme inhibitor enalapril in patients with normal left ventricular function and optimal beta blockade. J Am Coll Cardiol 2001; 37:470. Arnold AL, Milner KA, Vaccarino V. Sex and race differences in electrocardiogram use (the National Hospital Ambulatory Medical Care Survey). Am J Cardiol 2001; 88:1037.
142. Seils DM, Friedman JY, Schulman KA. Sex differences in the referral process for invasive cardiac procedures. J Am Med Womens Assoc 2001; 56:151.
143. Polk DM, Naqvi TZ. Cardiovascular disease in women: sex differences in presentation, risk factors, and evaluation. Curr Cardiol Rep 2005; 7:166.
144. Bairey Merz CN, Shaw LJ, Reis SE, et al. Insights from the NHLBI-Sponsored Women's Ischemia Syndrome Evaluation (WISE) Study: Part II: gender differences in presentation, diagnosis, and outcome with regard to gender-based pathophysiology of atherosclerosis and macrovascular and microvascular coronary disease. J Am Coll Cardiol 2006; 47:S21.
145. Mieres JH, Gulati M, Bairey Merz N, et al. Role of noninvasive testing in the clinical evaluation of women with suspected ischemic heart disease: a consensus statement from the American Heart Association. Circulation 2014; 130:350.
146. Orencia A, Bailey K, Yawn BP, Kottke TE. Effect of gender on long-term outcome of angina pectoris and myocardial infarction/sudden unexpected death. JAMA 1993; 269:2392.
147. Kannel WB, Vokonas PS. Demographics of the prevalence, incidence, and management of coronary heart disease in the elderly and in women. Ann Epidemiol 1992; 2:5.
148. Lerner DJ, Kannel WB. Patterns of coronary heart disease morbidity and mortality in the sexes: a 26-year follow-up of the Framingham population. Am Heart J 1986; 111:383.
149. Mosca L, Linfante AH, Benjamin EJ, et al. National study of physician awareness and adherence to cardiovascular disease prevention guidelines. Circulation 2005; 111:499.
150. Wenger NK. You've come a long way, baby: cardiovascular health and disease in women: problems and prospects. Circulation 2004; 109:558.
151. Alter DA, Naylor CD, Austin PC, Tu JV. Biology or bias: practice patterns and long-term outcomes for men and women with acute myocardial infarction. J Am Coll Cardiol 2002; 39:1909.
152. Michos ED, Vasamreddy CR, Becker DM, et al. Women with a low Framingham risk score and a family history of premature coronary heart disease have a high prevalence of subclinical coronary atherosclerosis. Am Heart J 2005; 150:1276. Taylor BC, Wilt TJ, Welch HG. Impact of diastolic and systolic blood pressure on mortality: implications for the definition of "normal". J Gen Intern Med 2011; 26:685.
153. Ahmed ME, Walker JM, Beevers DG, Beevers M. Lack of difference between malignant and accelerated hypertension. Br Med J (Clin Res Ed) 1986; 292:235.
154. Severe symptomless hypertension. Lancet 1989; 2:1369.
155. O'Mailia JJ, Sander GE, Giles TD. Nifedipine-associated myocardial ischemia or infarction in the treatment of hypertensive urgencies. Ann Intern Med 1987; 107:185.
156. Grossman E, Messerli FH, Grodzicki T, Kowey P. Should a moratorium be placed on sublingual nifedipine capsules given for hypertensive emergencies and pseudoemergencies? JAMA 1996; 276:1328.
157. Forman JP, Stampfer MJ, Curhan GC. Diet and lifestyle risk factors associated with incident hypertension in women. JAMA 2009; 302:401.
158. Sonne-Holm S, Sørensen TI, Jensen G, Schnohr P. Independent effects of weight change and attained body weight on prevalence of arterial hypertension in obese and non-obese men. BMJ 1989; 299:767.
159. Staessen JA, Wang J, Bianchi G, Birkenhäger WH. Essential hypertension. Lancet 2003; 361:1629.
160. Wang NY, Young JH, Meoni LA, et al. Blood pressure change and risk of hypertension associated with parental hypertension: the Johns Hopkins Precursors Study. Arch Intern Med 2008; 168:643.
161. Carnethon MR, Evans NS, Church TS, et al. Joint associations of physical activity and aerobic fitness on the development of incident hypertension: coronary artery risk development in young adults. Hypertension 2010; 56:49.
162. de Simone G, Devereux RB, Chinali M, et al. Risk factors for arterial hypertension in adults with initial optimal blood pressure: the Strong Heart Study. Hypertension 2006; 47:162. Colberg SR, Sigal RJ, Fernhall B, et al. Exercise and type 2 diabetes: the American College of Sports Medicine and the American Diabetes Association: joint position statement. Diabetes Care 2010; 33:e147.
163. American Diabetes Association. Standards of medical care in diabetes--2014. Diabetes Care 2014; 37 Suppl 1:S14.
164. Centers for Disease Control and Prevention (CDC). Dental visits among dentate adults with diabetes--United States, 1999 and 2004. MMWR Morb Mortal Wkly Rep 2005; 54:1181.
165. Inoue M, Iwasaki M, Otani T, et al. Diabetes mellitus and the risk of cancer: results from a large-scale population-based cohort study in Japan. Arch Intern Med 2006; 166:1871.
166. Stattin P, Björ O, Ferrari P, et al. Prospective study of hyperglycemia and cancer risk. Diabetes Care 2007; 30:561.
167. Hemminki K, Li X, Sundquist J, Sundquist K. Risk of cancer following hospitalization for type 2 diabetes. Oncologist 2010; 15:548.
168. Giovannucci E, Harlan DM, Archer MC, et al. Diabetes and cancer: a consensus report. Diabetes Care 2010; 33:1674.
169. Larsson SC, Mantzoros CS, Wolk A. Diabetes mellitus and risk of breast cancer: a meta-analysis. Int J Cancer 2007; 121:856.

170. Tsilidis KK, Kasimis JC, Lopez DS, et al. Type 2 diabetes and cancer: umbrella review of meta-analyses of observational studies. BMJ 2015; 350:g7607. Booth GL, Kapral MK, Fung K, Tu JV. Recent trends in cardiovascular complications among men and women with and without diabetes. Diabetes Care 2006; 29:32.

171. Vamos EP, Bottle A, Edmonds ME, et al. Changes in the incidence of lower extremity amputations in individuals with and without diabetes in England between 2004 and 2008. Diabetes Care 2010; 33:2592.

172. Pasquale LR, Kang JH, Manson JE, et al. Prospective study of type 2 diabetes mellitus and risk of primary open-angle glaucoma in women. Ophthalmology 2006; 113:1081.

173. Obrosova IG, Chung SS, Kador PF. Diabetic cataracts: mechanisms and management. Diabetes Metab Res Rev 2010; 26:172.

174. Centers for Disease Control and Prevention (CDC). Correctable visual impairment among persons with diabetes--United States, 1999-2004. MMWR Morb Mortal Wkly Rep 2006; 55:1169. Global Strategy for Asthma Management and Prevention, Global Initiative for Asthma (GINA). www.ginasthma.org (Accessed on January 30, 2015).

175. Standards for the diagnosis and care of patients with chronic obstructive pulmonary disease. American Thoracic Society. Am J Respir Crit Care Med 1995; 152:S77.

176. Siafakas NM, Vermeire P, Pride NB, et al. Optimal assessment and management of chronic obstructive pulmonary disease (COPD). The European Respiratory Society Task Force. Eur Respir J 1995; 8:1398.

177. BTS guidelines for the management of chronic obstructive pulmonary disease. The COPD Guidelines Group of the Standards of Care Committee of the BTS. Thorax 1997; 52 Suppl 5:S1.

178. Obstructive lung disease. Med Clin North Am 1990; 74:547.

179. Rosenbloom J, Campbell EJ, Mumford R, et al. Biochemical/immunologic markers of emphysema. Ann N Y Acad Sci 1991; 624 Suppl:7.

180. Petty TL, Silvers GW, Stanford RE. Mild emphysema is associated with reduced elastic recoil and increased lung size but NOT with air-flow limitation. Am Rev Respir Dis 1987; 136:867.

181. O'Brien C, Guest PJ, Hill SL, Stockley RA. Physiological and radiological characterisation of patients diagnosed with chronic obstructive pulmonary disease in primary care. Thorax 2000; 55:635.

182. Jeffery PK. Comparison of the structural and inflammatory features of COPD and asthma. Giles F. Filley Lecture. Chest 2000; 117:251S.

183. Castaldi PJ, San José Estépar R, Mendoza CS, et al. Distinct quantitative computed tomography emphysema patterns are associated with physiology and function in smokers. Am J Respir Crit Care Med 2013; 188:1083.

184. Hersh CP, Washko GR, Estépar RS, et al. Paired inspiratory-expiratory chest CT scans to assess for small airways disease in COPD. Respir Res 2013; 14:42.

185. Estépar RS, Kinney GL, Black-Shinn JL, et al. Computed tomographic measures of pulmonary vascular morphology in smokers and their clinical implications. Am J Respir Crit Care Med 2013; 188:231.

186. Aoshiba K, Nagai A. Differences in airway remodeling between asthma and chronic obstructive pulmonary disease. Clin Rev Allergy Immunol 2004; 27:35.

187. Baraldo S, Turato G, Badin C, et al. Neutrophilic infiltration within the airway smooth muscle in patients with COPD. Thorax 2004; 59:308.

188. Sutherland ER, Martin RJ. Airway inflammation in chronic obstructive pulmonary disease: comparisons with asthma. J Allergy Clin Immunol 2003; 112:819.

189. Turato G, Zuin R, Miniati M, et al. Airway inflammation in severe chronic obstructive pulmonary disease: relationship with lung function and radiologic emphysema. Am J Respir Crit Care Med 2002; 166:105.

190. Cosio MG, Saetta M, Agusti A. Immunologic aspects of chronic obstructive pulmonary disease. N Engl J Med 2009; 360:2445.

191. Hogg JC. Pathophysiology of airflow limitation in chronic obstructive pulmonary disease. Lancet 2004; 364:709.

192. Hogg JC, Chu F, Utokaparch S, et al. The nature of small-airway obstruction in chronic obstructive pulmonary disease. N Engl J Med 2004; 350:2645. Jia CE, Zhang HP, Lv Y, et al. The Asthma Control Test and Asthma Control Questionnaire for assessing asthma control: Systematic review and meta-analysis. J Allergy Clin Immunol 2013; 131:695.

193. Rank MA, Bertram S, Wollan P, et al. Comparing the Asthma APGAR system and the Asthma Control Test™ in a multicenter primary care sample. Mayo Clin Proc 2014; 89:917.

194. Osborne ML, Pedula KL, O'Hollaren M, et al. Assessing future need for acute care in adult asthmatics: the Profile of Asthma Risk Study: a prospective health maintenance organization-based study. Chest 2007; 132:1151.

195. Enright PL, Lebowitz MD, Cockroft DW. Physiologic measures: pulmonary function tests. Asthma outcome. Am J Respir Crit Care Med 1994; 149:S9.

196. Crapo RO. Pulmonary-function testing. N Engl J Med 1994; 331:25.

www.ingramcontent.com/pod-product-compliance
Lightning Source LLC
Chambersburg PA
CBHW072304200526
45168CB00014B/477